Making Sense of Evidence-based Practice for Nursing

T0262394

This straightforward guide to evidence-based practice helps you to develop the knowledge and skills necessary to challenge practice that is not underpinned by research and to increase your understanding of the processes involved in accessing, appraising, and synthesizing good quality research.

Providing a basic introduction to both quantitative and qualitative research, Debra Evans explores how to find out "what works best", the impact of something, and what requires more research. Readers will also learn the basic rules used in study design and statistics presented in research articles and systematic reviews. Each simply written chapter includes relevant theory, diagrams and tables, case studies, exercises, boxed summaries, and further reading.

Packed with examples from practice across the nursing fields and at different levels, this book is essential for nurses – both student and qualified – who want to increase their confidence when it comes to research appraisal and evidence-based practice processes.

Debra Evans is a senior lecturer at Birmingham City University, UK.

Making Sense of Evidence-based Practice for Nursing

An Introduction to Quantitative and Qualitative Research and Systematic Reviews

Debra Evans

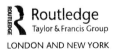
Routledge
Taylor & Francis Group

LONDON AND NEW YORK

Cover image: Getty Images

First published 2023
by Routledge
4 Park Square, Milton Park, Abingdon, Oxon OX14 4RN

and by Routledge
605 Third Avenue, New York, NY 10158

Routledge is an imprint of the Taylor & Francis Group, an informa business

© 2023 **Debra Evans**

British Library Cataloguing-in-Publication Data
A catalogue record for this book is available from the British Library

Library of Congress Cataloging-in-Publication Data
Names: Evans, Debra, Dr., author.
Title: Making sense of evidence-based practice for nursing : an introduction to quantitative and qualitative research and systematic reviews / Debra Evans.
Description: Abingdon, Oxon ; New York, NY : Routledge, 2022. | Includes bibliographical references and index.
Identifiers: LCCN 2022010587 (print) | LCCN 2022010588 (ebook)
Subjects: LCSH: Nursing—Research—Methodology. | Evidence-based nursing. | Evidence-based medicine.
Classification: LCC RT81.5 .E93 2022 (print) | LCC RT81.5 (ebook) | DDC 610.73072—dc23/eng/20220512
LC record available at https://lccn.loc.gov/2022010587
LC ebook record available at https://lccn.loc.gov/2022010588

ISBN: 978-0-367-74084-9 (hbk)
ISBN: 978-0-367-74083-2 (pbk)
ISBN: 978-1-003-15601-7 (ebk)

DOI: 10.4324/9781003156017

Illustration credit:
Rory Evans Birks

Contents

List of figures   vii
List of tables   ix
List of boxes   xii
Foreword   xv
Preface   xviii
Acknowledgements   xx
List of abbreviations   xxii

1   Introduction to research and evidence based practice   1

Step 1: Pose a focused research question   **11**

2   How do you put together a good focused research question?   13

Step 2: Search for the evidence   **23**

3   How do you search for evidence to answer that question?   25

Step 3: Critically appraise the evidence   **35**

4   When you have found some evidence how do you know if it's any good?   37

5 Let's talk about the characteristics of a quantitative
design – the randomised controlled trial   50

6 Some non-randomised quantitative designs – quasi
experiments, cohort studies and case-control studies   64

7 What are effect measures for dichotomous outcomes? 77

8 What are effect measures for continuous outcomes?   95

9 How do you critically appraise quantitative evidence
such as RCTs?   105

10 Let's talk about characteristics of some qualitative
designs – phenomenology, ethnography and
grounded theory   118

11 How do you critically appraise qualitative evidence? 132

Step 4: Making a decision to implement the evidence 145

12 Why we need systematic reviews and initiatives
like the Cochrane Library   147

13 Clinical guidelines and implementation of EBP   164

14 Your role in all of this?   173

Index   181

Figures

5.1	"Design" logo	50
5.2	"Rapid heal" RCT representation	53
5.3	Bias "bubbles" – to show where bias could have crept in	54
5.4	RCT features that improve design and minimise bias	55
5.5	"Honey" RCT representation	60
5.6	Bias "bubbles" – to show where bias could have crept in	61
6.1a	Exposed cohort	69
6.1b	With outcome	69
6.1c	Without outcome	69
6.1d	Not exposed cohort	69
6.1e	With outcome	69
6.1f	Without outcome	69
6.1g	Exposed	71
6.1h	Not exposed	71
6.1i	Cases with outcome	71
6.1j	Exposed	71
6.1k	Not exposed	71
6.1l	Controls without outcome	71
7.1	"Rapid heal" RCT representation	79
7.2	Follow me	83
7.3	Number line to show RR = 0.8 95% CI 0.4 to 1.2	88
7.4	Number line to show RR = 0.8 and 95% CI 0.7 to 0.9	91
8.1	"Rapid heal" RCT representation	95
8.2	Follow me	96
8.3	Number line to show MD = 1.3 95% CI –0.1 to 2.7	100
8.4	Number line to show MD = –2 95% CI –1.5 to –2.5	102

9.1	"Honey" RCT representation	107
10.1	"Design" logo	118
12.1	Primary studies	147
12.2	Systematic reviews	147
12.3	Number line to show RR = 0.8 95% CI 0.7 to 0.9	152
12.4	Number line to show RR = 0.8 95% CI 0.7 to 0.9	152
12.5	Number line to show RR = 0.7 95% CI 0.3 to 1.1	152
12.6	Number line to show RR = 0.7 95% CI 0.65 to 0.75	152
12.7	Forest plot	153

Tables

1.1	What this shift in thinking resulted in	2
1.2	Some differences between quantitative and qualitative research approaches	6
1.3	Questions from the different fields of nursing regarding **"is there a cause and effect"** relationship	7
1.4	Questions from the different fields of nursing regarding **"is there an association with"** relationship	7
1.5	Questions from the different fields of nursing regarding **"how someone feels"**	8
1.6	Steps in EBP	8
2.1	Step 1	13
2.2	Examples of a quantitative and a qualitative research question	14
2.3	PICOD table	15
2.4	PICOD table	16
2.5	PICOD table	17
2.6	PEO table	18
2.7	District nurse questions	19
2.8	Health visitor questions	20
2.9	Advanced nurse practitioner questions	20
3.1	Step 2	25
3.2	List of places to search for evidence	26
3.3	PICOD table	27
3.4	Demonstration of how the PICOD framework can be used to construct a basic search strategy	28

3.5   Questions from the different fields of nursing
      regarding **"is there a cause and effect"** relationship   28
3.6   Demonstration of how the PEO framework can be
      used to construct a basic search strategy   29
3.7   Questions from the different fields of nursing
      regarding **"how someone feels"**   29
3.8   Example search strategy for a district nurse question   30
3.9   Example search strategy for a health visitor question   31
3.10 Example search strategy for an advanced clinical
      practitioner question   32
4.1   Examples of topics of interest to a nurse   38
4.2   Different philosophical viewpoints   41
4.3   Example ACP question and search strategy   43
4.4   Example children's nurse question and search strategy   46
5.1   Basic steps in an RCT applied to hypothetical
      scenario$_1$ 51
5.2   Examples of **"what works best"** questions from the
      four nursing fields   57
5.3   ACP **"what works best"** question   57
5.4   Basic steps in an RCT applied to hypothetical scenario$_2$ 58
6.1   Examples of "is there an association with" question
      from the different nursing fields   72
6.2   The SIDS example as a potential case-control study   72
7.1   Hypothetical trial looking at fictitious "rapid heal"
      on chronic wounds summary   77
7.2 2×2 table   84
7.3 2×2 table   86
7.4   Questions from the different branches of nursing
      regarding "is there a cause and effect" relationship   88
7.5 2×2 table   89
7.6   Interpreting dichotomous measures of effectiveness   91
8.1   Interpreting continuous measures of effectiveness   102
9.1   Step 3   105
9.2   Summary of work done so far regarding the
      hypothetical "honey trial"   106
10.1 Some qualitative research approaches   119
10.2 Some qualitative data collection methods   120
10.3 Some qualitative data analysis methods   121

10.4	Basic steps in descriptive phenomenology applied to HYPOTHETICAL "scenario 1"	122
10.5	Quantitative and qualitative quality criteria	125
10.6	Examples of "how someone feels" questions from the four nursing fields	127
10.7	Children's nurse **"how does it feel"** question	127
10.8	Basic steps in descriptive phenomenology applied to HYPOTHETICAL "scenario 2"	127
10.9	Qualitative quality criteria	129
11.1	Step 3	132
11.2	Steps qualitative researchers can take for the different qualitative quality criteria	133
11.3	Summary of work done so far regarding the hypothetical "parents' perceptions" study	135
11.4	Basic steps in descriptive phenomenology applied to HYPOTHETICAL "scenario 2"	136
11.5	Qualitative quality criteria applied to qualitative "scenario 2"	137
12.1	What the systematic reviewers would do with included studies	151
12.2	Results from the three included studies in the hypothetical systematic review	152
12.3	Hypothetical forest plot to indicate how it might appear in a systematic review: comparison: honey vs. saline, outcome 1: mucositis (any) – so a dichotomous outcome	153
12.4	Questions from the different fields of nursing regarding "what works best"	156
12.5	Questions from the different fields of nursing regarding "how someone feels"	158
12.6	Similarities between the EBP processes and SR processes	159
13.1	A summarisation of the EBP, SR, and clinical guideline development processes	170
14.1	Steps you could take to be an evidence-based practitioner	174

Boxes

1.1   Common questions nurses ask   1
1.2   The need to include evidence   4
1.3   Hierarchy of designs   5
2.1   Focusing your question   14
2.2   Adult field example   15
2.3   Using the PICO structure to guide us, the focused
      research question would be . . .   15
2.4   Child field example   16
2.5   Using the PICO structure to guide us, the focused
      research question would be . . .   16
2.6   Mental health field example   17
2.7   Using the PICO structure to guide us, the focused
      research question would be . . .   17
2.8   Learning disabilities field example   18
2.9   Using the PIO/PEO structure to guide us, the focused
      research question would be . . .   18
4.1   Definition of health care research   37
4.2   Quantitative scenario   39
4.3   Qualitative scenario   40
4.4   ACP question answered by a quantitative approach
      to highlight this approach's characteristics and
      philosophical underpinnings   44
4.5   Children's nurse question answered by a qualitative
      approach to highlight this approach's characteristics
      and philosophical underpinnings   46

5.1	RCT definition	51
5.2	Steps that could be taken to minimise bias in scenario 1	56
5.3	Steps that could be taken to minimise bias in scenario 2	61
6.1	Quasi-experiments: description	67
6.2	Cohort studies: description	68
6.3	Case-control studies: description	70
6.4	Hypothetical case-control study exploring SIDS	73
7.1	Dichotomous outcomes	83
7.2	Hypothetical trial looking at the effect of "rapid heal" on healing and not healing wounds	84
7.3	Interpretation of RR	85
7.4	Interpretation of 95% CI	88
7.5	Hypothetical trial looking at the effect of honey on presence or absence of oral mucositis at 1 week	89
7.6	Interpretation of RR	90
7.7	Interpretation of 95% CI	90
8.1	Continuous outcomes	96
8.2	Hypothetical trial looking at the effect of "rapid heal" on the average reduction in wound surface area at 2 weeks	97
8.3	Interpretation of the mean difference	98
8.4	Interpretation of the 95% CI	99
8.5	Hypothetical trial looking at the effect of honey on the average pain score after 1 week	100
8.6	Interpretation of the mean difference	101
8.7	Interpretation of the 95% CI	101
9.1	Features the Consort document (Moher et al, 2010) states it is important to describe	109
10.1	Phenomenology definition	121
11.1	Features the COREQ document states it is important to clearly describe	139
12.1	Some milestones in relation to quantitative systematic reviews (cited by Chalmers et al, 2002 and Clarke, 2015)	149
12.2	Purposes quantitative systematic reviews can serve (Mulrow, 1994)	150

12.3	Included study 1	151
12.4	Milestones in relation to qualitative systematic reviews	156
12.5	Purposes qualitative systematic reviews may serve	157

Foreword

This is a welcome book for the nursing community and has been produced by an established and expert academic, Dr Debra Evans from Birmingham City University. Dr Evans has significant expertise in education, teaching research methods to undergraduate and postgraduate students.

It has long been a challenge within health care and health care courses to ensure that there is the ability to inculcate a significant amount of knowledge to students in a way that allows them to build skills and capability for future practice in evidence-based nursing. The theory–practice debate has long been a challenge within nursing, and many students find this a challenge. Importantly, research as a core topic, that is intrinsically part of a critical thinking practitioner, requires a great deal of time and thought to ensure that these concepts are taken on board by students not only for the completion of their programme, but for onward use as qualified practitioners and potentially for future research opportunities.

Dr Evans's book is a long-awaited addition to a wide range of support literature to students. However, Dr Evans has taken a different approach which is highly innovative and well-structured and poses a set of questions in a way that students will easily be able to relate to. This relatability is a key part of her engagement strategy with students so they are able to contextualise the approaches they may wish to take at the undergraduate level and, importantly, postgraduate level.

The structure of the chapters is extremely logical and takes the reader through a series of questions and approaches to build knowledge capability and learning. This text will certainly be integral to support modules in undergraduate and postgraduate programmes. It will also be a required reference text for many within practice who wish to review their approaches to evidence-based deployment alongside those who practice clinical teaching of students around evidence-based practice.

Dr Evans has focused significantly on a range of techniques within the writing that simplify some of the complex issues around evidence-based practice in a way that a range of students will be able to access and support their learning. Dr Evans uses a number of examples from clinical practice and teaching which really illuminate some of the more nuanced and technical discussions in relation to evidence-based practice. The use of summaries is extremely helpful to students to collate their learning from the individual chapters and also poses further questions in relation to how they relate this to their own studies or clinical work.

The references for each of the chapters are well developed and involve primary texts which are extremely important in study design, as well as more recent concepts, with more recent examples of how this has been applied in the clinical research setting.

There is particularly good use of visual tools within the text construction and chapters that really do help simplify some of the concepts to aiding understanding by students. These are peppered with real-life examples and questions to further aid students' understanding of evidence-based practice.

This new text is an ideal support to a wide range of health care professionals. However, it is primarily focused on nurses, but would have resonance with allied health professionals and midwives. It has been constructed in a way that makes it highly accessible as an entry-level text that gives a wide range of information on the full options in relation to research methods and evidence-based practice. This text is therefore aimed well at the undergraduate level, and for early career nurses is highly ideal and a welcome addition. This would also be a helpful aid memoir in clinical practice for those who are undertaking further work on internal practice or early career research.

I think Dr Evans has completed an extremely difficult task in producing a highly accessible textbook on evidence-based practice that will have great impact on a wide range of students. It is a welcome addition to the literature, and I am sure would be an important addition to reading lists on the majority of undergraduate and postgraduate nursing programmes.

Professor Mark Radford, PhD, RN
Chief Nurse, Health Education England
Deputy Chief Nursing Officer (England)

Preface

My experience has been that many excellent, motivated students have not looked forward to, or have been worried about, studying evidence-based practice (EBP) either due to the research language, the very comprehensive but weighty texts, a lack of statistical knowledge, or not seeing the relevance of different research approaches to their practice at first. I hope my attempt at helping you make sense of EBP will be challenging and encourage critical thinking – whilst at the same time not being so complicated it puts you off.

What do I think makes my book different? It's probably shorter than others. It contains recent examples of research questions important to nurses in all fields and specialities – many developed with my students – that will hopefully spark your interest. I have created hypothetical research questions in order to illustrate how common quantitative and qualitative research approaches and systematic reviews can be utilised and appraised to inform the evidence base. I have placed particular emphasis on quantitative research approaches related to determining the effectiveness of interventions – because nurses administer lots of interventions – and need to know what works best on a daily basis. I have tried to keep the writing style conversational with lots of illustrations, colour and worked examples. Similarly to how I teach it, I have tried to introduce concepts incrementally to help you get to grips with EBP in stages, so this book is designed to be read from Chapter 1 to Chapter 14.

I have over 20 years of experience trying to engage nursing and health care students with this topic on a weekly basis. I trained as a Registered General Nurse (RGN), have a quantitative scientific background from studying a PhD and a Degree in physiology, and professional recognition as an educator in higher education (Senior Fellow of the Higher Education Academy [SFHEA]). I completed a clinical trials course, a systematic review course, and a statistics course whilst working as a senior lecturer and subsequently was part of teams undertaking a clinical randomised controlled trial (RCT) and quantitative systematic reviews (SRs) for Cochrane. I tried to draw on these experiences and the evidence base to incorporate effective ways of teaching EBP when designing and delivering my master's- and degree-level core EBP, research methods and dissertation modules. Within those modules I have particularly focused on including the quantitative aspects, as previously, they had been under-represented in my place of work. You will hopefully see why this shift was important as you read the book.

With that in mind, this book will focus on getting you started with constructing focused clinical research questions; developing your search skills to find evidence; identifying and interpreting different types of evidence relevant to what you need to know; demonstrating competent skills in the appraisal of evidence, particularly the quantitative; describing, interpreting, and evaluating findings, again particularly the quantitative; and considering issues related to using this evidence to bring about practice change.

In summary, this book is not designed to replace existing in-depth texts, which, of course, I encourage you to read *after* this book. It is designed to initially interest and engage you in EBP in a straightforward, pragmatic way. To encourage you to "scratch the surface" of the evidence that underpins your practice, especially about "what works best". I'd like to think it will give you confidence and skills to challenge existing practice if required; to access, judge, and utilise evidence if possible; and, of course, to achieve the learning outcomes of core EBP, research methods and dissertation modules at the degree/master's level that you may be studying.

Acknowledgements

I want to acknowledge my students – not many people start out thinking they are going to be a lecturer in research methodology. I had the option to be a lecturer in physiology, but it turned out I made the right choice for me. Although having a career teaching about research methods doesn't sound too exciting, the many research ideas my students have had over the years have made my job "colourful". The range of topics from advanced nurse practitioners, professional practice nurses, health visitors, school nurses, district nurses, neonatal nurses, and nurses from all four fields of nursing have helped keep my job interesting and varied. I have enjoyed helping my students develop ideas into searchable questions or viable research endeavours. I have gained the most enjoyment from teaching students who initially struggled with this topic – as an educator, it is extremely rewarding when they say "It is starting to make sense".

I would like to acknowledge my colleagues – two in particular – Dr Phil Dee for being my critical friend, talking statistics and reading through early drafts of my quantitative chapters; and Dr Chris Inman for being my long-standing friend and colleague because when I was busy promoting the joys of quantitative research, she was there reminding me of the virtues of qualitative. I would also like to thank Dr Rob Cook for making me realise how difficult it is to explain confidence intervals correctly. I would also like to thank my friend and colleague, Lucy Land – between us in the late 1990s we bounced lots of ideas off each other and managed to get systematic reviews onto the curriculum for core EBP and research modules at our place of work. I would like to thank Stephen Gough and Helen Ryba, who helped me appreciate the nuances of searching for evidence with their technical expertise and who over the years have helped many of my students refine their search skills. I would also like to acknowledge Nathalie Turville for sharing my office – always a good friend, a good sounding board, and never once complained about my very poor commitment to washing up the coffee cups.

Last but not least my friends and family. Bernie, Mandy, and Sarah – who read chapters for me – and over the years have provided great friendship, meals out, trips to France, and laughs. My friends Gail and Tammy, who have listened to me go on about this book over many a walk or a cappuccino. My parents, who have always thought that education was important and have supported me in any educational endeavour. My sister, her partner, and my niece for hosting fun trips to Holland. And finally Matthew and my children, Dan, Rory, and Millie. Without Rory's quiet patience and technical skills, my sketches wouldn't have been turned into his much better digital drawings. Thanks also to Dan, Rory, and Millie for putting up with me saying for over a year "in a minute", "won't be long", "I've just got to save this". And thanks to Matthew for about 800 cups of tea and reminding me when I got side-tracked thinking, "Am I writing a methodology book?", "How much should I go into the statistics?", "Can I write such a book?" – that I wasn't trying to be some great academic; rather, I was trying to capture my experience of teaching this topic for many years and putting it into a book that might help students make sense of EBP.

Abbreviations

AGREE	Appraisal of Guidelines, Research and Evaluation
ANP	Advanced nurse practitioner
ASSIA	Applied Social Sciences Index and Abstracts
CASP	Critical Appraisal Skills Programme
CENTRAL	Cochrane Central Register of Controlled Trials
CHN	Community health nurse
CI	Confidence interval
CINAHL	Cumulative Index for Nursing and Allied Health
CONSORT	Consolidated Standards of Reporting Trials
COREQ	Consolidated criteria for reporting qualitative research
CQRMG	Cochrane Qualitative and Implementation Methods Group
DN	District nurse
DV	Dependent variable
EBHC	Evidence-based health care
EBP	Evidence-based practice
EPPI-centre	Evidence for Policy and Practice Information and Co-ordinating Centre
GDGs	Guideline development groups
GRADE	Grading of Recommendations, Assessment, Development and Evaluations
GRADE-CERequal	GRADE-Confidence in the Evidence from Reviews of Qualitative research

HV	Health visitor
IV	Independent variable
JBI	Joanna Briggs Institute
M_C	Mean of the control group
MD	Mean difference
M_E	Mean of the experimental group
NGC	National guideline centre
NH	Null hypothesis
NICE	National Institute for Health and Care Excellence
NIHR	National Institute for Health Research
NMC	Nursing and midwifery council
NRS	Non-randomised studies
O_C	Odds of the event in the control group
O_E	Odds of the event in the experimental group
OR	Odds ratio
PEO	Population, Exposure (to), Outcome
PICO	Population, Intervention, Counter-Intervention, Outcome
PICOD	Population, Intervention, Counter-Intervention, Outcome, Design
PRISMA	Preferred reporting items for SRs and meta-analyses
p-values	Probability values
QES	Qualitative evidence synthesis
QUOROM	Quality of reporting of meta-analysis statement
R_C	Risk of the event in the control group
RCT	Randomised controlled trial
R_E	Risk of the event in the experimental group
RH	Research hypothesis
ROB	Risk of bias
ROBiNRS	Risk of bias in non-randomised studies
RR	Risk ratio
SCPHN	Specialist community public health nurse
SIGN	Scottish Intercollegiate Guideline Network
SN	School nurse
SR	Systematic review
SRQR	The standards for reporting qualitative research

STROBE	The Strengthening the Reporting of Observational Studies in Epidemiology
TED	Technology, entertainment and design
TNP	Topical negative pressure
VAC	Vacuum-assisted wound closure
WHO	World Health Organization

1 Introduction to research and evidence-based practice

Introduction

Box 1.1 Common questions nurses ask

"Mmm . . . what works best? . . .

"How does that make someone feel"? . . .

This book will introduce you to how you can look at health care information in a more critical way. This should help you make more informed decisions about care you provide, or for that matter, care you receive. It will provide you with an overview of evidence-based practice (EBP) and teach you about the PROCESSES involved. It will hopefully act as a bridge or stepping-stone between you and more in-depth books on this topic.

What are health care interventions?

They could be for example:

Medication
Medical devices
Dressings
Topical agents
Alternative therapies
Psycho-social interventions
Educational interventions
Talking therapies

Topical agent

Medication

Dressing

DOI: 10.4324/9781003156017-1

Big questions to ask yourself

> How do you know if they work?
> Is one better than another?
> How does that make someone feel?
> Can you trust the claims?
> Who are the stakeholders?
> Who stands to benefit from the findings?
> Are there any ethical implications?
> "Research says . . ." – Does it?
> "The evidence suggests . . ." – Does it?

In the 1990s there was a shift in thinking regarding the education of initially medics regarding how clinical decisions were made in medicine (Dawes et al, 2005, Evidence-Based Medicine Working Group, 1992, Guyatt & Rennie, 1993). It used to be believed that clinical experience, intuition, logical reasoning, and knowledge of anatomy, physiology, and pathophysiology were sufficient to inform practice and guide decision making. History has shown us that they were not sufficient, on their own, to inform practice – an understanding of EVIDENCE/RESEARCH and how to access, judge, and incorporate it was required (Dawes et al, 2005, Guyatt & Rennie, 1993, Sackett et al, 1996, Sackett, 2000). This thinking filtered through into nursing (Mazurek Melnyk & Fineout-Overholt, 2005) and other health care professions. You only have to look at nursing degree and master's courses to see that EBP and research modules are now a core part of the curriculum so students can learn about evidence/research and how it can inform practice!

This shift in thinking was very beneficial

Table 1.1 What this shift in thinking resulted in

It meant more effective interventions and treatments being used
It resulted in more harmful interventions being stopped or withdrawn

This is an ongoing process

So what is EBP? There are various definitions which all emphasise that up-to-date, good-quality evidence must be incorporated into decision making – looking at it from either the care provider's or the care recipient's perspective:

> Evidence based medicine is the *conscientious, explicit, and judicious use of current best evidence* in making decisions about the care of individual patients. The practice of evidence based medicine means integrating individual clinical expertise with the best available external clinical evidence from systematic research.
>
> *(Sackett et al, 1996)*

> Evidence based public health is the *conscientious, explicit, and judicious use of current best evidence* in making decisions about the care of communities and populations in the domain of health protection, disease prevention, health maintenance and improvement.
>
> *(Jenicek, 1997)*

> Evidence-Based Practice (EBP) requires that decisions about health care are based on the *best available, current, valid and relevant evidence*. These decisions should be made by those receiving care, informed by the tacit and explicit knowledge of those providing care, within the context of available resources.
>
> *(Dawes et al, 2005)*

Box 1.2 The need to include evidence

If you are not convinced about the need to include evidence, here are some examples cited by Torgerson and Torgerson (in chapter 1 of their excellent book on designing RCTs in health, education, and the social sciences) of health care disasters when "treatments" or interventions were *not* first evaluated by any *or* the most appropriate research (Torgerson & Torgerson, 2008, pp. 1–8):

- 1940s and 1950s – administration of oxygen to premature babies
- 1940s and 1950s – administration of prophylactic antibiotics to premature babies
- 1980s – "routine" use of antiarrhythmia drugs for patients post-myocardial infarction
- 2000s – "standard" therapy of high-dose steroids for patients with head injuries

Listen to Ben Goldacre's TED talk on tackling "Bad Science", which includes more examples of interventions that don't work or even do harm (Goldacre, 2011).

To add to that the Nursing and Midwifery Council (NMC) states that "nurses should always practise in line with the best available evidence and to achieve this must make sure that any information or advice given is evidence-based, including information relating to using any health and care products or services and maintain the knowledge and skills needed for safe and effective practice" (Nursing and Midwifery Council, 2021).

Clinical decision making

So in addition to clinical experience, RESEARCH EVIDENCE must also be incorporated into health care decision making. It is also important that patient preferences and resources be taken into account (DiCenso et al, 1998, Haynes et al, 1996, Sackett et al, 1996).

So what does evidence look like?

Hierarchy of evidence

As this heading suggests, there exists a ranking of the types of evidence, with some considered better than others (Canadian Task Force on the Periodic Health Examination, 1979, Sackett, 1989).

If you want to know "what works best" in a health care scenario – a question posed earlier – current thinking is that you would be better using evidence higher up the hierarchy. Why, you may ask at this point?

It is to do with the idea that more is built into the research designs to reduce bias the higher up the hierarchy you go, which increases the internal validity of the study – but more on this later.

The designs in this hierarchy are referred to as QUANTITATIVE

> **Box 1.3   Hierarchy of designs**
>
> Quantitative hierarchy of evidence
> Something at the top
> Something at the bottom
> As you go up the hierarchy, **BIAS** decreases
> So as you go up the hierarchy, **INTERNAL VALIDITY** increases

DESIGNS – again more on that later. At the top is **systematic reviews** (SRs) – this is known as secondary research because rather than the researcher doing his or her own randomised controlled trial (RCT), he or she systematically reviews other people's RCTs on a specific intervention. Below that are the primary studies – the **randomised controlled trial**, then **quasi-experiments**, then **cohort studies**, then **case-control studies**, then case series and case reports, right down to expert opinion (Canadian Task Force on the Periodic Health Examination, 1979, Sackett, 1989).

Don't worry if you aren't familiar with these designs – we will go through them in later chapters.

If you want to know "how someone feels" or their experience of some phenomena or some circumstance in a health care scenario – another question posed earlier – you need different evidence obtained through primary QUALITATIVE DESIGNS (e.g. phenomenology). There are **SRs** of qualitative research too. Again, don't worry if you aren't familiar with these designs – we will go through them in later chapters.

Table 1.2 Some differences between quantitative and qualitative research approaches

Quantitative	Qualitative
At its most basic interpretation, students often understand quantitative research to mean it generates numbers and statistics which from my experience immediately puts a lot of students off – but it is much more than that.	At its most basic interpretation, students understand qualitative research to mean it generates narrative and words – but it is much more than that and has a totally different purpose from quantitative research.
Quantitative researchers often want to determine if there is some type of relationship between two variables e.g. is there a relationship between the type of dressing you might use for a wound and the rate of healing? This relates to "what works best" if you had two dressings to choose from.	Qualitative researchers often want to explore a phenomena in its entirety e.g. the experience of having a chronic wound that doesn't heal. This relates to "how does it feel" if you had patients with non-healing chronic wounds.
Basically, quantitative research is often about:	Basically, qualitative research is often about:
• Testing hypotheses to see if there are relationships between variables	• Generating theories
• There is lots of control and measurement – depending on how much – determines whether you can establish <u>causation</u> or just <u>association</u> between variables	• There is little control and no measurement, the aim being to look at some phenomena holistically (Polit & Beck, 2018, p. 18)
• It measures outcomes, which generate numbers and use statistics	• It often generates narrative and observations and looks for patterns, themes, and concepts
• It seeks to generalise findings from relatively large random samples to a target population	• It seeks to provide credible descriptions or interpretations of some phenomena that is context bound – and involves relatively small, purposive samples
• There is an empirical basis for generalising quantitative findings, meaning that, through observation and experiment, hypotheses are validated or refuted	• There is a "theoretical rather than an empirical basis for generalising from qualitative findings" (Ploeg, 2008, p. 56)

(Continued)

Table 1.2 (Continued)

Quantitative	Qualitative
• It contributes to the evidence base by finding out if there are relationships between variables and therefore can help determine "what works best".	• It contributes to the evidence base by enriching someone's understanding of such a phenomena and might help illuminate "how does it feel" for those individuals

So I hope that gives you a little flavour of what quantitative and qualitative research/evidence can achieve when well conducted. We will look at both approaches in a lot more detail later on.

For now let's focus on what sort of evidence you require as a user/consumer of it in order to make better health care decisions.

The sort of evidence/research you need depends on the question you want to answer

Table 1.3 Questions from the different fields of nursing regarding "is there a cause and effect" relationship

Adult field example: Does **topical negative pressure** heal chronic wounds?	Child field example: Does **emollient cream** resolve childhood eczema?
Mental health field example: Do **coping strategies** reduce stress in carers of relatives with dementia?	Learning disabilities field example: Does **exercise** reduce anxiety in people with a learning disability?

Regarding the "what works best" question posed earlier, to answer these, you need systematic reviews of RCTs (quantitative) or if there isn't one, RCTs.

Table 1.4 Questions from the different fields of nursing regarding "is there an association with" relationship

Adult field example: Is there an association between vaping and lung disease?	Child field example: Is there an association between passive smoking and children's health?
Mental health field example: Is there an association between eating disorders and osteoporosis?	Learning disabilities field example: Is there an association between socioeconomic background and accessing support services?

Looking forward in time or looking back in time, is/was there an association with a particular intervention or exposure to something and a particular outcome? To answer these, you need quantitative cohort studies (prospective) or case-control studies (retrospective).

Table 1.5 Questions from the different fields of nursing regarding "how someone feels"

Adult field example: What is the impact of a non-healing venous leg ulcer in adults?	Child field example: What is the impact of repeated surgeries in children?
Mental health field example: What is the impact of repeated miscarriages in women?	Learning disabilities field example: What is the impact of caring for a child with profound multiple learning disabilities on family carers?

What is the impact of a condition, an experience, treatment, or intervention on an individual? – the "how someone feels" question posed earlier – to answer these you need systematic reviews of qualitative studies or if there isn't one – individual qualitative studies.

So how do you go about giving the best care? You need to learn about and then apply the five-step EBP process (Sackett et al, 1996).

Table 1.6 Steps in EBP

Steps	EBP process
PICOD PICO PEO	1. Pose a focused research question
	2. Search for the evidence
	3. Critically appraise the evidence
✗ OR ✓	4. Make a decision to implement the evidence (or not) alongside your clinical experience, patients' preferences, and resources
	5. Evaluate this

Summary

- Not all practice in health care professions is evidence-based.
- In the past experience, intuition and logical reasoning were used to underpin practice.
- In some instances this led to withholding of effective treatments and continuing with harmful interventions.
- Current thinking does not disregard experience, intuition, and reasoning but recognises that evidence is also required to underpin practice.
- However, not all evidence is equally trustworthy or equally unbiased.
- The sort of evidence that is appropriate depends on the research question being asked.
- If it is to try to establish the relationship between variables or to find out **"what works best"**, quantitative approaches are often used.
- If it is to try to establish the impact of some phenomena or circumstance on someone to find out **"how does it feel"**, qualitative approaches are often used.
- An evidence-based practitioner needs to familiarise themselves with the processes of asking the right question; searching for, appraising, synthesizing, and deciding whether to integrate the evidence into the clinical decision; and then evaluating it.

References

Canadian Task Force on the Periodic Health Examination. (1979) The periodic health examination. *The Canadian Medical Association Journal*; 121: 1193–1254.

Dawes M, Summerskill W, Glasziou P. et al. (2005) Sicily statement on evidence-based practice. BMC *Medical Education*; 5: 1. doi: 10.1186/1472-6920-5-

DiCenso A, Cullum N, Ciliska D. (1998) Implementing evidence-based nursing: Some misconceptions. *Evidence-Based Nursing*; 1: 38–39.

Evidence-Based Medicine Working Group. (1992) Evidence-based medicine. A new approach to teaching the practice of medicine. JAMA; 268: 2420–2425.

Goldacre B. (2011) Ben Goldacre: Battling bad science. *TED Talk*. Accessed on 05/10/2021.

Guyatt GH, Rennie D. (1993) Users' guides to the medical literature. JAMA; 270: 2096–2097.

Haynes RB, Sackett DL, Gray JM, Cook DJ, Guyatt GH. (1996) Transferring evidence from research into practice: 1. The role of clinical care research evidence in clinical decisions. *ACP Journal Club*; *125*(3) November–December: A14–16. PMID: 8963526.

Jenicek M. (1997) Epidemiology, evidence-based medicine, and evidence-based public health. *Journal of Epidemiology and Community Health*; 7: 187–197.

Mazurek Melnyk B, Fineout-Overholt E. (2005) *Evidence-Based Practice in Nursing and Health Care. A Guide to Best Practice*. Philadelphia, PA: Lippincott Williams & Wilkins.

Nursing and Midwifery Council. (2021) *The Code: Professional Standards of Practice and Behaviour for Nurses and Midwives*. The Code: Professional standards of practice and behaviour for nurses, midwives and nursing associates – The Nursing and Midwifery Council (nmc.org.uk). Accessed on 05/10/2021.

Ploeg J. (2008) Identifying the best research design to fit the question. Part 2: Qualitative research. In Cullum N, Ciliska D, Haynes RB, Marks S (Eds) *Evidence Based Nursing: An Introduction* (p. 56). Oxford: Blackwell Publishing Ltd.

Polit DF, Beck CT. (2018) *Essentials of Nursing Research: Appraising Evidence for Nursing Practice*. 9th edn. Philadelphia: Wolters Kluwer.

Sackett DL. (1989) Rules of evidence and clinical recommendations on the use of antithrombotic agents. *Chest*; 95: 2S–4S.

Sackett DL. (2000) *Evidence-based Medicine. How to Practice and Teach EBM* (p. 136). New York: Churchill Livingstone Inc.

Sackett DL, Rosenberg WM, Gray JA, Haynes RB, Richardson WS. (1996) Evidence based medicine: What it is and what it isn't'. *BMJ (Clinical Research Ed.)*; *312*(7023): 71–72.

Torgerson DJ, Torgerson CJ. (2008) Chapter 1: Background to controlled trials. In *Designing Randomised Trials in Health, Education and the Social Sciences* (pp. 1–8). Houndmills, Basingstoke, Hampshire: Palgrave Macmillan.

Step 1

Pose a focused research question

PICOD PICO PEO	

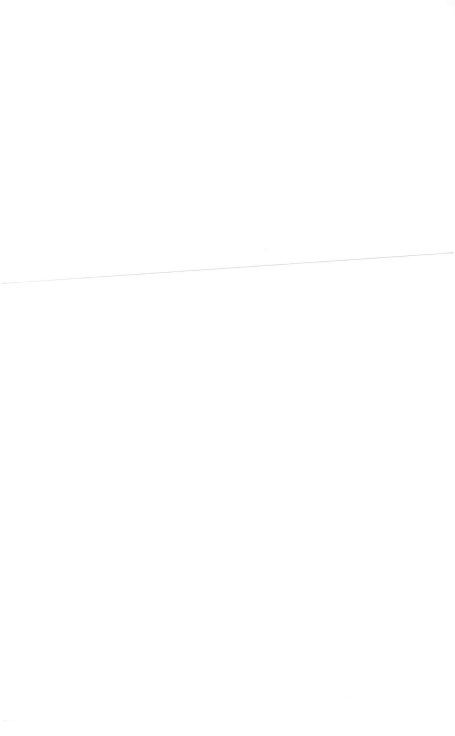

2 How do you put together a good, focused research question?

Table 2.1 Step 1

PICOD PICO PEO	1. Pose a focused research question

In this chapter I want to help you generate questions that arise from practice that you might want an answer to in order to best care for your patient group.

You will learn about the PROCESS of putting a clear, focused research question together using a framework. You will learn why these frameworks are useful when you are reading other people's research too in quickly identifying what is being studied and which research design it is likely to be employing.

Each time you learn about an EBP process, e.g. how to generate a focused research question using a framework, I will illustrate it with an example.

I will walk you through an exercise so you can apply what you have learned.

Generating the question

Following on from the previous chapter, try to think of a research question that arises from practice to see if you are clear about quantitative and qualitative research questions. Sometimes it is useful to use a mind map (Buzan, 1991) so you can identify an area of interest and its many facets then narrow down to specific aspects. As a starting point, it is helpful to reflect on your and others' practice and to

DOI: 10.4324/9781003156017-3

think if there are areas where you are not sure about an intervention's effectiveness or its impact. Being familiar with existing research will help you identify gaps in knowledge and a potential need for research.

Table 2.2 Examples of a quantitative and a qualitative research question

What is the effect of larval therapy on debriding sloughy wounds?	QUANTITATIVE – "what works best" question
How do patients feel about having larval therapy?	QUALITATIVE – "how does it feel" question

The process of putting a focused research question together using a framework

Several authors have suggested various frameworks and tools that can be used to put a focused research question together that gets you to think of the main important elements or frames the key search terms (McKibbon & Marks, 2001 Richardson et al, 1995). The well-known mnemonic **PICO** (Population, Intervention, Control/Counter-intervention, and Outcome) is widely cited and is designed to shape quantitative research questions (Counsell, 1997, Fineout-Overholt & Johnston, 2005, Straus et al, 2005). Sometimes D is added to denote the research design you would focus on looking for, such as RCTs (O'Connor et al, 2008). The PIO or **PEO** (Population, Exposure to, and Outcome)/PICo (Population, Interest in, and Context) format is designed to shape qualitative research questions (Kestenbaum, 2019). Usually in qualitative research questions there is no Control/Counter-intervention because the researcher is not seeking to compare an intervention with something else, but rather to seek valid accounts from individuals.

Box 2.1   Focusing your question

You need to identify five, four, or three things depending on the type of question:

PICOD

1. Who you are interested in
Population
2. What it is you are interested in
Intervention/Issue/Interest in/Exposure to

3. What you are interested in it being compared against
Counter-intervention
4. Which outcome(s) you are interested in
Outcome
5. What design best answers the question
Design

Example 1

Imagine you want to know how best to treat a chronic wound and you have heard about topical negative pressure (TNP). How do you turn that into a focused research question that you can search for evidence on? Ask yourself:

Who is the Population of interest?
What is the Intervention of interest (usually the newer product in this case)?
What is the Counter-intervention?
What is the Outcome(s) of interest?
What Design best answers the question?

Table 2.3 PICOD table

Population	Intervention	Counter-intervention	Outcome	Design
Adults with chronic wounds	Topical negative pressure	No treatment/ sham/alternative Treatment	Wound healing	SR or RCT

So instead of . . .

Box 2.2   Adult field example

Does topical negative pressure heal chronic wounds?

Box 2.3   Using the PICO structure to guide us, the focused research question would be . . .

"In adults with chronic wounds, what is the effect of topical negative pressure compared to no treatment/sham/alternative treatment on wound healing?" A "what works best – is there a cause and effect" type question best answered with an SR of RCTs or an RCT.

Example 2

Imagine you want to know how best to treat childhood eczema and you have come across lots of different creams, including emollients. How do you turn that into a focused research question that you can search for evidence on? Ask yourself:

Who is the Population of interest?
What is the Intervention of interest (emollient in this case)?
What is the Counter-intervention?
What is the Outcome(s) of interest?
What Design best answers the question?

Table 2.4 PICOD table

Population	Intervention	Counter-intervention	Outcome	Design
Children	Emollient	Alternative product	Resolution of eczema	SR or RCT

So instead of . . .

Box 2.4　Child field example

Does emollient cream resolve childhood eczema?

Box 2.5　Using the PICO structure to guide us, the focused research question would be . . .

"In children with eczema, what is the effect of emollient cream compared to alternative products on resolving this skin condition?" Another "what works best – is there a cause and effect" type question best answered with a systematic review of RCTs or an RCT.

Example 3

Imagine you have heard that in young women with eating disorders, there is a potential association with osteoporosis. How do you turn this into a focused research question to find out more? Ask yourself:

Who is the Population of interest?
What is the Intervention of interest/Issue (eating disorder in this case)?
What is the Counter-intervention?
What is the Outcome(s) of interest?
What Design best answers the question?

Table 2.5 PICOD table

Population	Intervention/ Issue	Counter-intervention	Outcome	Design
Female adolescents	Eating disorder	No eating disorder	Bone mineral density	Cohort or case-control designs

So instead of . . .

Box 2.6   Mental health field example

Is there an association between eating disorders and osteoporosis?

Box 2.7   Using the PICO structure to guide us, the focused research question would be . . .

"In female adolescents, how does having an eating disorder compare with not having an eating disorder on bone mineral density?" An "is there an association" type question best answered with a quantitative cohort study design or a case-control design.

Example 4

Imagine in this scenario you wanted to know how to best support family carers looking after a child with profound multiple learning disabilities. How do you turn this into a focused research question? Ask yourself:

Who is the Population of interest?
What is the Interest in/Exposure to (having a child with profound multiple learning disabilities)?
What is the Outcome(s) of interest (the family carers' experiences)?
What Design best answers the question?

Table 2.6 PEO table

Population	Interest in/Exposure to	Outcome	Design
Family carers	Child with profound multiple learning disabilities	Experience	Qualitative

So instead of . . .

Box 2.8   Learning disabilities field example

What is the impact of caring for a child with profound multiple learning disabilities on family carers?

Box 2.9   Using the PIO/PEO structure to guide us, the focused research question would be . . .

"When family carers take care of a child with profound multiple learning disabilities, what are their experiences?" This is a "how does it feel" type question best answered with an SR of qualitative studies or, if absent, a qualitative study design.

From these four examples, I hope you can see how PICO (or PICOD) or PIO (sometimes referred to as PEO) frameworks ensure a focused research question, making it very clear to the reader all the important elements of the research (McKibbon & Marks, 2001, Richardson et al, 1995). In the next chapter you will see how these frameworks can be used to create very useful search strategies to look for research to answer these questions.

So to reiterate, creating a PICO or PIO/PEO framework helps with the **FIRST** step of the EBP process, which is to **construct a focused research question,** and it can be used to construct search strategies which help inform the **SECOND step** of the EBP process, which is to **search for the research on that topic**. We will consider how to search effectively in greater detail in the next chapter.

To make sure you have understood these frameworks, have a go at identifying the PICO or the PIO/PEO from the following research questions generated by **community health nurses, specialist community public health nurses**, and **advanced nurse practitioners** I have taught. Look at the research question being asked and ask yourself if it is a "what works best" type question, thus requiring quantitative research to answer it, or a "how does it feel" type question, thus requiring qualitative research to answer it. Have a go yourselves before looking at the sample answers.

Table 2.7 District nurse questions

District nurse (DN) question:
In adults with type 1 diabetes, on multiple daily injections, what is the effect of the FreeStyle Libre flash glucose monitoring system compared to capillary blood glucose monitoring on adherence in glucose testing?
Answer:
P   Adults living with type 1 diabetes on multiple daily insulin injections I   FreeStyle Libre flash glucose monitoring system C   Capillary blood glucose monitoring O   Adherence in glucose testing D   This is a "what works best" type question requiring randomised controlled trials (RCTs) to answer it
DN question:
Are male partners' health beliefs affected by female partners who are on a community-based programme aimed at reducing the incidence of falls in the elderly?
Answer:
P   Men E   Women attending a community-based programme aimed at reducing the incidence of falls in the elderly O   Health beliefs D   This is a "how does it feel" type question requiring qualitative studies, usually ones that have interviewed participants, to answer it

Table 2.8 Health visitor questions

Health visitor (HV) question:
In infants with a cleft palate what is the effect of Gaviscon, compared to other interventions, on the symptoms of colic?

Answer:

P	Infants with cleft palate with colic
I	Gaviscon
C	White noise, holding the baby through the crying episode or gentle motion, bathing in warm water, other winding techniques
O	Length of crying, colicky crying time, and fulfilment of colic criteria
D	This is a "what works best" type question requiring RCTs to answer it

HV question:
Are health visitors' attitudes towards victims of domestic abuse in their care affected by personal exposure to and experience of domestic abuse?

Answer:

P	Health visitors
E	Personal exposure to and experience of domestic abuse
O	Attitudes towards victims of domestic abuse in their care
D	This is a "how does it feel" type question requiring qualitative studies, usually ones that have interviewed participants, to answer it

Table 2.9 Advanced nurse practitioner questions

Advanced nurse practitioner (ANP) question:
With qualified nurses, what is the effect of high-fidelity simulation (HFS) training in deteriorating patient scenarios in comparison to alternative training methods on nurses' knowledge, skill performance, and self-confidence?

Answer:

P	Qualified nurses
I	HFS training in deteriorating patient scenarios
C	Traditional didactic lecture, traditional clinical training, or low- or medium-fidelity simulation
O	Nurses' knowledge, skill performance, and self-confidence
D	This is a "what works best" type question requiring RCTs to answer it

ANP question:
In adults diagnosed with type 2 diabetes mellitus advised to make dietary changes, what are the perceived barriers/experiences to making these changes?

(Continued)

Table 2.9 (Continued)

Answer:	
P	Patients age 18 years and up diagnosed with type 2 diabetes
E	Advised to make dietary changes after education
O	Barriers/experiences to making dietary changes
D	This is a "how does it feel" type question requiring qualitative studies, usually ones that have interviewed participants, to answer it

Summary

- Ideas for research questions come from all sorts of different sources – from you; from colleagues; from your patients, clients, family members, or carers; from issues arising from practice and your field of nursing; and, of course, from gaps in existing research.
- The first step of EBP is the process of putting a clear, focused research question together that is aided by the use of frameworks such as PICO and PIO/PEO.
- Once the question is in one of these formats, the EBP practitioner can use it to construct a search strategy to look for evidence and research, which we will consider in more detail in the next chapter.
- As an aside – when reading other people's research, it is very useful to quickly identify the PICO or PIO/PEO from the title or abstract, as it helps identify the important elements of the research and usually quickly indicates if it is a quantitative or qualitative piece of research.

References

Buzan T. (1991) *Using Both Sides of Your Brain*. 3rd edn. London: Penguin Books.

Counsell C. (1997) Formulating questions and locating primary studies for inclusion in systematic reviews. *Annals of Internal Medicine*; *127*: 380–387.

Fineout-Overholt E, Johnston L. (2005) Teaching EBP "asking searchable, answerable, clinical questions". *Worldviews Evid Based Nursing*; *2*: 157–160.

Kestenbaum B. (2019) General considerations in epidemiological research. In *Epidemiology and Biostatistics: An Introduction to Clinical Research*. 2nd edn. Cham: Springer Nature.

McKibbon KA, Marks S. (2001) Posing clinical questions: Framing the question for scientific inquiry. *AACN Clinical Issues*; *12*(4): 477–481.

O'Connor D, Green S, Higgins JPT. (2008) Chapter 5: Defining the review question and developing criteria for including studies. In Higgins JPT, Green S (Eds) *Cochrane Handbook of Systematic Reviews of Interventions*. Chichester: John Wiley & Sons.

Richardson WS, Wilson MC, Nishikawa J, Hayward RS. (1995) The well-built clinical question: A key to evidence-based decisions. *ACP Journal Club*; *123*: A12–A13.

Straus SE, Richardson WS, Glasziou P, Haynes RB. (2005) *Evidence-based Medicine: How to Practice and Teach EBM*. 3rd edn. Edinburgh; New York: Elsevier/Churchill Livingstone.

Step 2

Search for the evidence

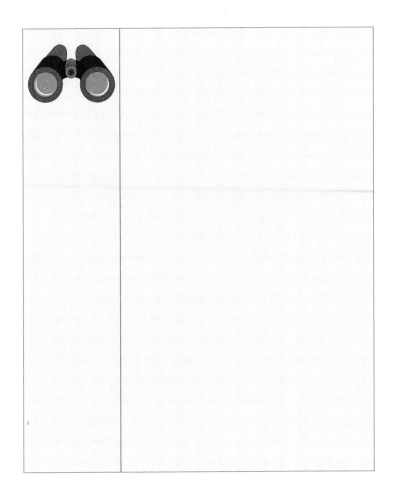

3 How do you search for evidence to answer that question?

Table 3.1 Step 2

	2. Search for the evidence

In this chapter, I want to help you find good-quality evidence to answer questions that arise from practice. You will learn that there are many places you can look for evidence. You will learn about the PROCESS of constructing a search strategy using the PICO or PIO/PEO framework and will start to consider why it is useful to look for **all** the evidence (published and unpublished, English and non-English, completed and ongoing) (Easterbrook et al, 1991, Egger et al, 1997, Haddaway et al, 2015).

Where to look for evidence

As hinted at in the first chapter, not all evidence is equally trustworthy, and when making decisions about health care, it is better to try to find the best evidence. This is usually in the form of quantitative and qualitative research studies, either pooled (in the form of systematic reviews) or individual, but you need to know where to find that. The *Cochrane Handbook* gives a very detailed section on where to search for evidence (Lefebvre et al, 2008).

DOI: 10.4324/9781003156017-5

Table 3.2 List of places to search for evidence

The Cochrane Library	This is the first place I tell my students to look if they have questions about "what works best". It has systematic reviews of RCTs looking at the effectiveness of health care interventions (remember I said this was top of the quantitative hierarchy of evidence for determining "what works best").
General health care databases (international)	Medline, Embase, and CENTRAL (Cochrane's central register of controlled trials) – CENTRAL is the best place to look for randomised controlled trials (RCTs), as it contains trials from the other two databases and other sources too (Lefebvre et al, 2008) (remember this is second from the top of the quantitative hierarchy of evidence for "what works best").
Subject-specific databases	Some examples: For nursing and allied health, there is Cumulative Index for Nursing and Allied Health (CINAHL). For social sciences and education, there is Applied Social Sciences Index and Abstracts (ASSIA). On these you will find both quantitative and qualitative research.
Citation indexes	Scopus – lists published articles known as "source articles" and links them to articles in which they have been cited. It is a way of searching forward in time (Lefebvre et al, 2008).
Dissertations/theses	EThOS – The UK's national theses service houses UK doctoral research theses.
Grey literature databases	Opensigle – For studies not formally published in journal articles but still important e.g. unpublished trials that did not show a difference in treatments – very important to know if you want the full picture.
Journals	Hand-searching. Full-text journals available electronically e.g. PubMed Central.
Conference abstracts/ proceedings	On the BIOSIS database, Web of Science, and psycINFO.

(Continued)

Table 3.2 (Continued)

Unpublished/ongoing studies	ClinicalTrials.gov.
National and international trial registers	All Trials.gov – International initiative led by Ben Goldacre to try to get "all trials registered, all results reported".
Trial results registers	

The process of constructing a search strategy

Let's consider using PICOD for how we would search such databases for evidence **in adults with chronic wounds on the effect of topical negative pressure compared to no treatment/sham/alternative treatment on wound healing**.

Table 3.3 PICOD table

Population	*Intervention*	*Counter-intervention*	*Outcome*	*Design*
Adults with chronic wounds	Topical negative pressure	No treatment/sham/ alternativetreatment	Wound healing	SR or RCT

When thinking about searching for good-quality evidence, you need to think about the alternative terms that can be used to describe the same concepts. WHY? Because you might miss out important research that is called topical negative pressure (TNP), for example, or something else.

Synonyms – topical negative pressure, vacuum-assisted wound closure

Acronyms – TNP (topical negative pressure), VAC (vacuum-assisted wound closure)

Plural/singular forms – wound, wounds

There are also **spelling variations, variations of root words, and wild cards** – the asterisk symbol "*" acts as a wildcard e.g. wound* will retrieve documents containing wound or wounds.

In addition, some electronic databases can help identify the most appropriate terms and any alternatives by having a thesaurus of preferred terms (Bramer et al, 2018, Khan et al, 2001).

Boolean operators

You can combine search terms using the words AND, OR, NOT, NEAR, and NEXT (Bramer et al, 2018, Khan et al, 2001, Straus et al, 2005).

OR. If you use OR between search terms, you will get documents containing at least one of those terms. This helps **expand** the search.

AND. If you use AND between search terms, you will only get documents that contain each of the terms specified. This helps **restrict** the search (Booth et al, 2016).

Table 3.4 Demonstration of how the PICOD framework can be used to construct a basic search strategy

Population	Intervention	Counter-intervention	Outcome	Design
#1 Adults with chronic wounds **OR** Non-healing wounds	#2 Topical negative pressure **OR** TNP **OR** Vacuum-assisted wound closure **OR** VAC	No treatment/ sham/alternative treatment	Wound healing	#3 SR **OR** RCT

#1 **AND** #2 **AND** #3 would provide a specific basic search strategy for evidence on TNP and chronic wounds in adults from appropriate research designs that consider "what works best".

Have a go at constructing PICODs and search strategies for these three examples.

Table 3.5 Questions from the different fields of nursing regarding "is there a cause and effect" relationship

Adult field example: The TNP was the adult field example which I did with the students together	Child field example: Does emollient cream resolve childhood eczema?
Mental health field example: Do coping strategies reduce stress in carers of relatives with dementia?	Learning disabilities field example: Does exercise reduce anxiety in people with a learning disability?

In a similar way, the PIO/PEO frameworks can also be used to construct search strategies.

Let's consider using PEO for how we would search such databases for evidence on **how to best support family carers looking after a child with profound multiple learning disabilities based on their experiences.**

Table 3.6 Demonstration of how the PEO framework can be used to construct a basic search strategy

Population	Exposure	Outcome	Design
#1 Family carers **OR** Parents **OR** mother **OR** father **OR** siblings **OR** relative	#2 Child with profound multiple learning disabilities	#3 Experience	Qualitative

#1 **AND** #2 **AND** #3 would provide a specific basic search strategy for evidence on family carers' experiences of caring for a child with profound multiple learning disabilities from appropriate research designs that consider "how does it feel".

Have a go at constructing search strategies using PEO for these three examples.

Table 3.7 Questions from the different fields of nursing regarding "how someone feels"

Adult field example: What is the impact of a non-healing venous leg ulcer in adults?	Child field example: What is the impact of repeated surgeries in children?
Mental health field example: What is the impact of repeated miscarriages in women?	Learning disabilities field example: The family carers' experiences of looking after a child with profound multiple learning disabilities was the learning disabilities field example which I did with the students together

I can appreciate this process looks somewhat daunting, but I want you to see that searching for evidence is an involved process. It is more than just looking at what you do, what has been done before, what your colleagues or experts say, and what happened to one or two people. There is a wealth of information in the form of research to be found in places like the databases and journals noted earlier.

Employing specific search strategies improves your chances of finding appropriate research for your research questions to aid decision making (Eriksen & Frandsen, 2018). Faculty librarians are skilled information retrievers. In my place of work, they have been instrumental and key in facilitating both students and staff in conducting successful searches.

The results of searches can be saved in programs such as Endnote, Procite, Refman, and Refworks (Lefebvre et al, 2008).

Later on we will look into the problems associated with language and publication bias, but for now have a think about if you would have ALL the evidence if you only accessed English articles and published articles?

Have a go at constructing a search strategy with the PICO or PEO examples from **community health nurses, specialist community public health nurses**, and **advanced nurse practitioners** I have taught. I have provided sample answers, but have a go yourselves before looking.

Remember the purpose of this is to try to maximize your chances of finding relevant research to answer your research question and not to miss any relevant studies.

Table 3.8 Example search strategy for a district nurse question

DN question:
In adults with long-term indwelling urethral or suprapubic catheters, does triclosan, when compared to sterile water, affect encrustation and blockages and pain related with catheter changes?

Answer:

P	Adults over the age of 18 with an indwelling or suprapubic catheter
I	Triclosan solution or Farco-fill Protect
C	Standard intervention of sterile water
O	Encrustation and blockages and pain related with catheter changes
D	This is a "what works best" type question requiring RCTs to answer it

(Continued)

Table 3.8 (Continued)

Sample search strategy answer:				
P	I	C	O	D
#1 Adults with Catheters **OR** Urinary catheter **OR** Suprapubic catheter **OR** Indwelling catheter	#2 Triclosan **OR** Farco-fill Protect **OR** Farco-fill **OR** Antimicrobial blocking solution	Sterile water	Encrustation **OR** Blockages **OR** Pain	#3 SR **OR** RCTs

#1 **AND** #2 **AND** #3 would provide a specific basic search strategy for evidence on triclosan solution (and any other names for it) for adults with a catheter (and any other terms for catheter) from appropriate quantitative research designs that consider "what works best – is there a cause and effect relationship".

Table 3.9 Example search strategy for a health visitor question

HV question:
In infants under 1, is there an association between soft bedding and sudden infant death syndrome (SIDS) cases?

Answer:

P	Infants
I	Soft bedding
C	Non-soft bedding
O	Rates of SIDS
D	This is an "is there an association" type question usually referring to cohort studies or case-control studies to explore it

Sample search strategy answer:				
P	I	C	O	D
#1 Bab* **OR** Infant* **OR** Under 1 years old **OR** Newborn	#2 Soft bedding **OR** Soft blanket **OR** Duvet **OR** Quilt **OR** Pillow	Non-soft bedding	#3 Sudden infant death rates **OR** SIDS rates **OR** Cot death rates	Cohort **OR** Case-control studies

#1 **AND** #2 **AND** #3 would provide a specific basic search strategy for evidence on soft baby sleeping products (and any other names for them) for infants under 1 (and any other terms for babies) from appropriate quantitative research designs that consider is there an association with/or looking back was there an association with bedding type and SIDs rates.

Table 3.10 Example search strategy for an advanced clinical practitioner question

ACP question:			
In adults with long-term conditions who attend nurse-led clinics, what are their experiences in relation to self-management of such conditions?			

Answer:

P	Adults aged over 18 with a long-term condition
E	Nurse-led clinic
O	Experience in relation to self-management
D	This is a "how does someone feel" type question requiring qualitative studies, usually ones that have interviewed participants, to answer it

Sample search strategy answer:			
P	I/E	O	D
#1 Adults with long-term condition **OR** Adults with chronic illness **OR** Adults with chronic disease	#2 Nurse-led clinic **OR** Nurse-managed clinic **OR** Nurse clinic	#3 Experience in relation to self-management	Qualitative

#1 **AND** #2 **AND** #3 would provide a basic search strategy for evidence on patients' experiences in relation to self-management of a long-term condition having attended nurse-led clinics, usually looking at appropriate qualitative research designs that consider "how does it feel".

Although these are simplified basic search strategies, I hope it has started to convey the process involved in a "searching for evidence" task. Please do refer to more in-depth books on the topic.

Summary

- A wealth of places can be searched for good-quality evidence.
- Search strategies can be used to search these electronic databases.
- The EBP practitioner can use frameworks such as PICO and PIO/PEO to construct a search strategy.
- Alternative terms might be synonyms, acronyms, plural/singular forms, spelling variations, variations of root words, and wild cards.

- Some electronic databases can help identify the most appropriate terms and any alternatives by having a thesaurus of preferred terms.
- Boolean operators such as OR and AND can be used to expand or restrict the search.
- Even then, searches can still suffer from language or publication bias.

References

Booth A, Sutton A, Papaioannou D. (2016) *Systematic Approaches to a Successful Literature Review.* 2nd edn. London: Sage.

Bramer WM, de Jonge GB, Rethlefsen ML Mast F, Kleijnen J. (2018) A systematic approach to searching: An efficient and complete method to develop literature searches. *Journal of the Medical Library Association: JMLA; 106*(4): 531–541. doi: 10.5195/jmla.2018.283

Easterbrook PJ, Berlin JA, Gopalan R, Matthews DR. (1991) Publication bias in clinical research. *Lancet; 337:* 867–872.

Egger M, Zellweger-Zähner T, Schneider M, Junker C, Lengeler C, Antes. (1997) Language bias in randomised controlled trials published in English and German. *Lancet; 350:* 326–329.

Eriksen MB, Frandsen TF. (2018) The impact of patient, intervention, comparison, outcome (PICO) as a search strategy tool on literature search quality: A systematic review. *Journal of the Medical Library Association: JMLA; 106*(4): 420–431.

Haddaway NR, Collins AM, Coughlin D. et al. (2015) The role of Google scholar in evidence reviews and its applicability to grey literature searching. *PlOS ONE; 10*(9): 1–17. Imp of grey lit

Khan KS, ter Riet G, Glanville J, Soweden AJ, Kleijnen J (eds) (2001) *Undertaking Systematic Reviews of Research on Effectiveness: CRD's Guidance for Those Carrying Out or Commissioning Reviews* (CRD report number 4). 2nd edn. York (UK): NHS centre for reviews and dissemination. University of York.

Lefebvre C, Manheimer E, Glanville J. (2008) Chapter 6: Searching for studies. In Higgins JPT, Green S (eds) *Cochrane Handbook of Systematic Reviews of Interventions* (p. 129). Chichester: John Wiley & Sons.

Straus SE, Richardson WS, Glasziou P, Haynes RB. (2005) *Evidence-based Medicine: How to Practice and Teach EBM.* 3rd edn. Edinburgh; New York: Elsevier/Churchill Livingstone.

Step 3

Critically appraise the evidence

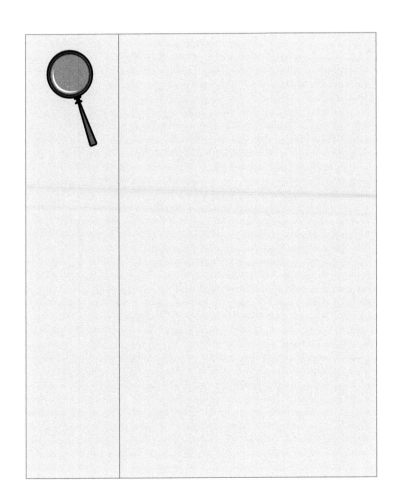

4 When you have found some evidence, how do you know if it's any good?

So far with regard to EBP we have begun to consider the process of how to put a good, focused question together and the process of how to search for evidence about this. The next step with EBP is the PROCESS of how to **critically appraise** the evidence or research found. But before you can do this, we need to spend the next eight chapters learning about what this means.

Critical appraisal is the process of "carefully and systematically examining research to judge its trustworthiness, and its value and relevance in a particular context" (Burls, 2009).

But you may ask, what do you need to examine to know if the research is TRUSTWORTHY?

Let's first consider how health research differs from anecdote, for example.

Box 4.1   Definition of health care research

Health research entails systematic collection or analysis of data with the intent to develop generalizable knowledge to understand health challenges and mount an improved response to them.

(WHO, 2021)

Let us think again about things of interest a health care professional might want to understand or study further.

DOI: 10.4324/9781003156017-7

Table 4.1 Examples of topics of interest to a nurse

"What works best – is there a cause and effect" questions	Adult field example: Does **topical negative pressure** heal chronic wounds?	Child field example: Does **emollient cream** resolve childhood eczema?
	Mental health field example: Do **coping strategies** reduce stress in carers of relatives with dementia?	Learning disabilities field example: Does **exercise** reduce anxiety in people with a learning disability?
"Is there an association" questions	Adult field example: Is there an association between vaping and lung disease?	Child field example: Is there an association between passive smoking and children's health?
	Mental health field example: Is there an association between eating disorders and osteoporosis?	Learning disabilities field example: Is there an association between socioeconomic background and accessing support services?
"How does it feel" questions	Adult field example: What is the impact of a non-healing venous leg ulcer in adults?	Child field example: What is the impact of repeated surgeries in children?
	Mental health field example: What is the impact of repeated miscarriages in women?	Learning disabilities field example: What is the impact of caring for a child with profound multiple learning disabilities on family carers?

We can see that areas of interest to nurses and health care professionals are diverse; you may be interested in lots of people or a few, adults or children; whether some intervention is effective or whether exposure to some factor is associated with some outcome; or the impact of some experience or circumstances on someone.

If you were a biomedical scientist, you might be predominantly interested in the relationship between variables, so mainly utilise randomised controlled trials (quantitative approaches). If you were a sociologist, you might be predominantly interested in meaning when studying social trends and mainly utilise qualitative research.

Your job as a nurse is a difficult one because when considering providing best care for your patients, your interests may span a range of research questions across several disciplines like physiology, psychology, and sociology. Because of this, you need to understand a range of research approaches that tend to inform these areas, rather than just one.

It is helpful to consider what guides a researcher when undertaking ANY TYPE of health care research. A researcher is guided by **the research process** (Polit & Beck, 2018) which consists of:

1. The conceptual phase. This is where the researcher "sets the scene" as to why the research needs to be done and leads up to the purpose of the research.
2. The design and planning phase. This is where the researcher selects a research design to best answer the research question/purpose.
3. The data collection phase. This is where the researcher decides how the data will be collected. It may be quantitative or qualitative depending on the research question/purpose.
4. The analytic phase. This is where the researcher analyses the quantitative or qualitative data to try to answer the research question.
5. The dissemination phase. This occurs when the researcher writes up the study and tries to get it published.

I now want to run through a couple of scenarios to show you how different research questions can be answered by different research approaches but still follow the research process.

Box 4.2   Quantitative scenario

Consider again the research question "In adults with chronic wounds, what is the effect of topical negative pressure compared to no treatment/sham/alternative treatment on wound healing?" and use the research process as a guide.

1. We are seeking to establish the effectiveness of an intervention, to try to establish cause and effect, or to test a hypothesis.

▼

2. Use a **randomised controlled trial (RCT)/experimental** approach which is characterized by random sampling of participants, random assignment of participants to the experimental or control/comparison group, manipulation of the independent variable/intervention, measurement of the dependent variable/outcome, and control over extraneous (other) variables (DiCenso et al, 2005, Polgar & Thomas, 2008, Polit & Beck, 2018, Torgerson & Torgerson, 2008).

   ▼

3. Collect data through structured observation using a measuring instrument which must be valid and reliable.

   ▼

4. Analyse the **quantitative** data.

   ▼

5. Disseminate the findings.

Here I am trying to show you that a "what works best" research question requires an RCT to answer it and how an RCT **follows the research process**. From this brief overview, you can see this quantitative research design has certain characteristics that we will explore in more detail later on.

Box 4.3   Qualitative scenario

Consider again the research question "When family carers take care of a child with profound multiple learning disabilities, what are their experiences?" and use the research process as a guide.

1. We are seeking to describe and explore, possibly generate a theory, or gain insight into a situation or problem concerning a small number of individuals (intensive).

   ▼

2. Use a **qualitative** approach, which is characterised by the study of phenomena in its natural context, with no attempt to exert control over the situation, and the sample employed is often purposive (Astin & Long, 2014, DiCenso et al, 2005, Holloway & Galvin, 2016, Polit & Beck, 2018).

   ▼

3. Collect data through semi-/unstructured interviews, observation, or document analysis. The data must be **credible, transferable, dependable, and confirmable**.

▾

4. Analyse the **qualitative** data.

▾

5. Disseminate the findings.

Here I am trying to show you that a "how does it feel" research question requires a qualitative research approach to answer it and how such an approach **follows the research process too**. From this brief overview, you can see that this too has certain characteristics (very different from a quantitative approach) that we will explore in more detail later on.

So far we have been LED by the research question and GUIDED by the research process, and now I would like to make you AWARE of philosophical underpinnings informed by Polit and Beck (2018), Scotland (2012), and Taber (2013). This is to do with thinking about how we come to have knowledge of the world and different research approaches may have different underpinnings.

Table 4.2 Different philosophical viewpoints

How a positivist thinks . . .	How an interpretivist thinks . . .
"Reality exists; there is a real world driven by real, natural causes" (Polit & Beck, 2018, p. 7)	"Reality is multiple and subjective and mentally constructed by individuals" (Polit & Beck, 2018, p. 7)
Wants to understand the underlying causes of natural phenomena	Interested in the entirety of some phenomenon
Believes in objective reality	"The researcher interacts with those being researched so subjectivity and values are inevitable" (Polit & Beck, 2018)
The causes that drive things can be uncovered	
"Is associated with 'scientific' approaches" (Taber, 2013)	"Involves the researcher making sense of research participants' responses in relation to the research purposes" (Taber, 2013.)

(Continued)

Table 4.2 (Continued)

How a post-positivist thinks . . .	How a critical theorist thinks . . .
"All observation, including objective reality, is fallible" (Taber, 2013) Still seek objectivity but try to minimise any biases "Appreciate the barriers to knowing reality with certainty and seek probabilistic evidence" instead (Polit & Beck, 2018, p. 7) "Scientific knowledge is provisional in the sense that it is open to review in the light of new evidence" (Taber, 2013) "Knowledge is tentative, hypotheses are not proved but simply not rejected" (Creswell, 2009, p. 7)	"Knowledge is both socially constructed and influenced by power relations from within society" (Scotland, 2012, p. 13) The critical paradigm seeks to address issues of social justice and marginalism "Dig beneath the surface of social life and uncover the assumptions that keep human beings from a full and true understanding of how the world works" (Scotland, 2012, p. 13)

Bunniss and Kelly (2010) assert that "there is no one superior research approach within the research paradigms; all are valid and informative when used sensitively in context to answer an appropriate research question". So perhaps if you want to know "what works best" and to generalise, look for quantitative research (preferably RCTs), which often fits within the post-positivist way of thinking. If you want to know "how someone feels", look for qualitative research, which often positions itself within the interpretive, and sometimes the critical theory, way of thinking.

When you read quantitative or qualitative research articles, you will see they both follow the research process in the way they are written up – with a background section reflecting the conceptual phase of why the research needs to be undertaken and essentially "setting the scene"; a methodology section reflecting the research design/approach to be used that best answers the research question, which also includes consideration of how data was to be collected and analysed and underpinned with a certain philosophy; then a results section reflecting how the collected data (could be quantitative or qualitative) was analysed; this is usually followed by a discussion section comparing results with previous research and any study limitations; the production and publication of the research article reflects the dissemination phase.

To make sure you have understood, refer to the research questions posed by **community health nurses, specialist community public health nurses, and advanced nurse practitioners.**

You have already considered the research question being asked by them and asked yourself if it is a "what works best" type question, thus requiring quantitative research to answer it, or a "how does it feel" type question, thus requiring qualitative research to answer it.

You have also started to consider the search strategies required to search comprehensively for appropriate evidence. Now I want you to imagine the searches have been carried out and research has been found.

Start to think of the characteristics of the quantitative or qualitative research that might be found to see if you can start to appreciate how they have different characteristics and underpinning philosophies whilst also seeing how it applies to **community health nurses', specialist community public health nurses', and advanced nurse practitioners'** research interests.

Table 4.3 Example ACP question and search strategy

ACP question:	
In adults with radiation-induced oral mucositis, what is the effect of honey compared to 0.9% saline rinse on the presence or absence of oral mucositis and pain score?	
P	Adult patients with radiation-induced oral mucositis
I	Pure natural honey rinse
C	Routine mouth care by 0.9% saline rinse
O	The presence or absence of oral mucositis, pain score
D	This is a "what works best" type question requiring quantitative RCTs to answer it

(*Continued*)

Table 4.3 (Continued)

Sample search strategy:				
P #1 Adults with radiation therapy **OR** Radiotherapy **OR** Radiation induced oral mucositis	I #2 Honey **OR** Topical honey **OR** Natural honey **OR** Pure natural honey **OR** Honey rinse	C Saline rinse	O Presence of oral mucositis **OR** Pain score	D #3 SR **OR** RCTs

#1 **AND** #2 **AND** #3 would provide a basic search strategy for evidence on honey (and any other names for it) for adult patients with radiation-induced oral mucositis (and any other terms for it) from appropriate research designs that consider "what works best".

In truth, the search strategy would be more complex than this, but I have kept it simple just to illustrate this example.

Imagine you have now found a relevant **quantitative study** – a trial/RCT using your search strategy – and you are starting to look at the characteristics and underpinning philosophy of this quantitative research design.

Box 4.4   ACP question answered by a quantitative approach to highlight this approach's characteristics and philosophical underpinnings

1. The authors of the (HYPOTHETICAL) trial have sought to **establish the effectiveness** of honey; or to establish if honey has an effect on mucositis that is different from 0.9% saline; or to test a hypothesis, e.g. if honey is used, then it will have a different effect from 0.9% saline on the presence of oral mucositis and pain score.

   ▼

2. They have used an **RCT/experimental** approach, which is characterised by random sampling of adult patients with radiation-induced oral mucositis, RANDOM ASSIGN-MENT of participants, to the experimental (pure natural honey rinse) or control/comparison (0.9% saline rinse) group (this means leaving it purely to chance who receives honey and who receives 0.9% saline). This is the manipulation of the independent variable/intervention, and researchers have measured the dependent variables/outcomes – in this case,

the presence or absence of oral mucositis and pain score in both groups of participants, and tried to control extraneous (other) variables.

3. They have collected data through structured observation using a measuring instrument, which must be **valid and reliable** – in this case, for both groups of participants, looking for the presence or absence of oral mucositis and measuring pain using a valid and reliable pain assessment tool.

4. They have analysed the **quantitative** data by comparing the presence or absence of oral mucositis and pain scores in both groups of participants.

5. They have disseminated the findings by getting the work published, and this is the RCT that you have found from your searching.

Here I am trying to show you that a "what works best" research question requires a quantitative RCT to answer it and how an RCT follows the **research process**. From this **brief** overview, you can see it has certain characteristics that we have explored a little with the "honey as an intervention for oral mucositis" example.

A word about ethics – think about the ethical considerations of this study. When you were reading a study such as this, you would check if it had gained ethical approval – you would want to check if informed consent was sought and if the comparison group of participants received the most current evidence-based intervention for oral mucositis and this is what the honey was compared with. You would want to see if stopping guidance had been built in if one intervention during early analysis outperformed the other.

So to sum up, at this point you have seen how to pose a question using PICOD, construct a search strategy, and started to look at the characteristics of quantitative designs such as RCTs that your search might find. This is necessary before you can embark on the third step of the EBP process, which is to **critically appraise** such studies.

Table 4.4 Example children's nurse question and search strategy

Children's nurse question:
What are parents' perceptions of non-pharmacological strategies for managing their children's pain post-elective surgery?

P	Parents
E	Non-pharmacological strategies for their child
O	Perception in relation to managing their children's pain post-elective surgery
D	This is a "how does someone feel" type question requiring qualitative studies, usually ones that have interviewed participants, to answer it

Sample search strategy answer:

P #1 Parents **OR** Carers	I/E #2 Child **AND** Non-pharmacological interventions **OR** Play **OR** Distraction **OR** Controlled breathing **OR** Cognitive behaviour therapy **OR** Parental comforting	O #3 Experience in relation to it managing children's pain post-elective surgery	D Qualitative

#1 **AND** #2 **AND** #3 would provide a basic search strategy for evidence on parents' perceptions in relation to management of children's pain post-elective surgery, looking at appropriate research designs that consider "how does it feel".

Imagine you have now found a relevant **qualitative study** using your search strategy and you are looking at the characteristics and underpinning philosophy of this qualitative research design.

Box 4.5   Children's nurse question answered by a qualitative approach to highlight this approach's characteristics and philosophical underpinnings

1. The authors of the (HYPOTHETICAL) qualitative study have sought to **describe and explore** parents' perceptions of non-pharmacological interventions for managing their children's pain post-elective surgery and gain insight into a situation or problem concerning a small number of individuals (intensive).

▼

2. They have used a **qualitative** approach, which is character-
    ised by the study of phenomena in its natural context, with
    no attempt to exert control over the situation, and the sample
    employed is often purposive – so they have sought views and
    perceptions from a small number of parents whose children
    have had non-pharmacological interventions.

3. They have collected data through semi-/unstructured inter-
    views in this example using open-ended questions to explore
    parents' perceptions of it managing their children's pain post-
    elective surgery. The data must be **credible, transferable,
    dependable, and confirmable**.

4. They have analysed the **qualitative** data by trying to identify
    themes from the narrative.

5. They have disseminated the findings by getting the work pub-
    lished, and this qualitative study is one that you have found
    from your searching.

Here I am trying to show you that a "how does it feel" research
question requires a qualitative research approach to answer it
and how such an approach follows the research process. From this
brief overview, you can see that this too has certain characteristics (very different from a quantitative approach) that we have
explored in more detail in this "perceptions of non-pharmacological interventions" example.

A word about ethics – think about the ethical considerations
of this study, e.g. was ethical approval sought to interview these
parents, and when asking parents to open up about a potentially
upsetting experience, what support mechanisms were in place?

So to sum up, at this point you have seen how to pose a question
using PIO/PEO, construct a search strategy, and started to look at
the characteristics of a qualitative design that your search might
find. This is necessary before you can embark on the third step of
the EBP process, which is to **critically appraise** such studies.

Summary

- Before you can critically appraise evidence that you find, you have to understand why well-conducted research is more trustworthy than anecdote, for example.
- If research is done properly, it is systematic, rigorous, and ethical.
- Different research approaches and designs exist to answer different research questions.
- Even if it is a quantitative or qualitative design, it still follows the research process.
- Different research designs have different characteristics and philosophical underpinnings, which would be useful to familiarise yourself with.
- By beginning to understand these characteristics and design features, you will start to see if the research does or does not have them, making it more or less trustworthy.
- Grasping this is the start of developing your critical appraisal skills.

References

Astin F, Long A. (2014) Characteristics of qualitative research and its application. *British Journal of Cardiac Nursing*, 02; 9(2): 93–98.

Bunniss S, Kelly DR. (2010) Research paradigms in medical education research. *Medical Education*; 44(4): 358–336.

Burls A. (2009) *What is Critical Appraisal?* The Bandolier Report. http://www.bandolier.org.uk/painres/download/whatis/What_is_critical_appraisal.pdf?msclkid=2ee70a20bdfe11ecaff1d5d9317b676b

Creswell JW. (2009) *Research Design: Qualitative and Mixed Methods Approaches.* London: SAGE.

DiCenso A, Guyatt G, Ciliska D. (2005) *Evidence Based Nursing: A Guide to Clinical Practice.* St Louis, MO: Elsevier Mosby.

Holloway I, Galvin K. (2016) *Qualitative Research in Nursing and Healthcare.* John Wiley & Sons, Incorporated. *ProQuest Ebook Central.* https://ebook-central.proquest.com/lib/bcu/detail.action?docID=4622920.

Polgar S, Thomas SA. (2008) *Introduction to Research in the Health Sciences.* 5th edn. Edinburgh: Churchill, Livingstone.

Polit DF, Beck CT. (2018) *Essentials of Nursing Research: Appraising Evidence for Nursing Practice.* 9th edn. Philadelphia. Wolters Kluwer.

Scotland J. (2012) Exploring the philosophical underpinnings of research: Relating ontology and epistemology to the methodology and methods of the scientific, interpretive, and critical research paradigms. *English Language Teaching;* 5(9). doi: 10.5539/elt.v5n9p9

Taber KS. (2013) *Classroom-based Research and Evidence-based Practice: An Introduction.* 2nd edn. London: Sage.

Torgerson DJ, Torgerson CJ. (2008) Chapter 1: Background to controlled trials. In *Designing Randomised Trials in Health, Education and the Social Sciences* (pp. 1–8). Houndmills, Basingstoke, Hampshire: Palgrave Macmillan.

WHO. (2021) www.who.int/westernpacific/health-topics/health-research. Accessed on 31/10/2021.

5 Let's talk about the characteristics of a quantitative design – the randomised controlled trial

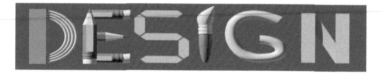

Figure 5.1 "Design" logo

As I said in the previous chapter, if you understand the characteristics of a research approach/design, you will better understand different research studies' methodological strengths and weaknesses. If you can recognise these strengths and weaknesses, you can start to appreciate how to critically appraise studies. This important skill helps you judge whether a study's findings are trustworthy or not and aids decision making. Ask yourself whether you trust the results. Would it lead to a change in practice?

Before you can learn about the PROCESS of appraising **quantitative** research studies, you need to learn about different quantitative research designs.

In previous chapters, I have already mentioned that if we want to know "what works best" or to try to establish cause and effect, it would be best to have the quantitative design randomised controlled trial (RCT). Remember that quantitative studies attempt to study large random samples of people and generalise to a target population. In this chapter we will focus on the **RCT**.

DOI: 10.4324/9781003156017-8

> ### Box 5.1 RCT definition
>
> RCTs are considered the best primary research design if you want to see "what works best". Put more formally, "RCTS are considered the most effective research design for determining which drugs, devices or procedures have superior diagnostic, therapeutic or prophylactic effectiveness" (US National Library of Medicine, 2008).

As I want to develop your critical thinking skills, we are still going to critically examine this claim. But first let me teach you about the basic setup of an RCT with this hypothetical scenario evaluating a **fictitious** dressing we shall call "rapid heal".

Scenario 1 – A research group has been asked to evaluate if a new dressing called "rapid heal" helps chronic wounds heal faster than other treatments in patients over 65 years of age. The manufacturers will pay for the study and at the end pay for a member of the research group to go to a wound conference to present the findings. The research group sees this is a "what works best" type of research question best answered by an RCT and proceeds to set up the trial.

Table 5.1 Basic steps in an RCT applied to hypothetical scenario₁

Remember I said earlier that with quantitative studies such as RCTs, it was about testing hypotheses. So the researcher proposes a research hypothesis (RH), which is designed to support a hunch. Often implicit is a null hypothesis (NH), which seeks to nullify the hunch (Henkel, 1976).	RH: If adults >65 with a chronic wound are given "rapid heal", then the healing rate will be different from those given an alternative treatment. (Note that I said different rather than better. Ethically, one should only conduct an RCT if there is **uncertainty** over what works best – "rapid heal" could make the healing rate worse.) NH: If adults over 65 with chronic wounds are given "rapid heal", then the healing rate will NOT be different from those given an alternative treatment and any observed difference will be due to chance.
Decide the intervention (I) and the counter-intervention (C).	I: "Rapid heal" dressing. C: Alternative dressing based on best available evidence.
Determine how the effect of I or C on the outcome (O) will be measured.	Measure how many wounds remain unhealed or have healed after 6 weeks. Compare the average reduction in wound surface area after 2 weeks.

(Continued)

Table 5.1 (Continued)

Identify the target population and select a random sample of people from it (P).	Following obtaining ethical approval (which includes stopping guidance), carry out the trial at several sites and hospitals that have adults over 65 with a chronic wound. Randomly select 200 patients to try to obtain a representative sample. Explain the purpose of the study, its benefits, any risks, and the voluntary nature of taking part before obtaining their written informed consent. Take some baseline measurements.
Randomly allocate half of the sample to I and half to C.	Leave it to chance of how patients of varying health and nutritional status are allocated to the two groups to create two groups, each containing 100 patients, that are hopefully balanced in terms of varying health and nutritional status (variables within an individual that might affect the outcome are called INTRINSIC variables).
Try to ensure constancy of conditions for both I and C groups.	Give the same care such as diet, turning schedules, same timings, and nurses doing dressing changes so both groups of participants are treated the same apart from whether they receive I or C (variables external to the individual that might affect the outcome are called EXTRINSIC variables).
Collate scores.	Measure in both groups of patients: 1. How many wounds have remained unhealed or healed after 6 weeks 2. The average reduction in wound surface area after 2 weeks
Analyse scores.	Compare groups using an appropriate statistical approach – if using hypothesis testing and p values (Wilkinson, 2013): If $p \leq 0.05$, it means the probability of getting the observed difference if chance was the only process operating (Gates, 2016) is very small ($<5\%$), so we reject the NH. If $p > 0.05$, it means the probability of getting the observed difference if chance was the only process operating (Gates, 2016) is more than 5% – that's considered too big so we are unable to reject the NH.
Say if can reject the NH or if unable to reject the NH (Campbell & Stanley, 1963, Wilkinson, 2013).	If we can reject the NH, the findings are said to be statistically significant. If we are unable to reject the NH, the findings are said to be not statistically significant.

Some students I have taught have found find it easier to picture the basic RCT setup with the following diagram (note the PICO), with "P" being the population of people over 65 with a chronic wound, "I" being the "rapid heal" dressing, "C" being the alternative dressing, and "O" being the healing outcome defined as the number of wounds remaining unhealed or healed after 6 weeks and the average reduction in wound surface area at 2 weeks:

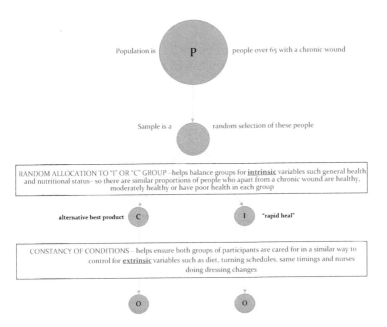

Figure 5.2 "Rapid heal" RCT representation

1. Outcome 1 compared how many wounds have remained unhealed and healed after 6 weeks.
2. Outcome 2 compared the average reduction in wound surface area at 2 weeks.

Let's imagine that when outcomes (O) are compared, the group that received "rapid heal" ("I") had fewer **unhealed** wounds

> at 6 weeks compared to the alternative dressing group ("C") and the statistical test said p <0.05, meaning the probability of getting such a difference between the groups, if chance was the only process operating, is very small (less than 5%), so you could reject the NH and say this was a statistically significant finding. You might be tempted to conclude that the "rapid heal" dressing "works best" – right? Not necessarily . . .

Fallible human beings carry out RCTs (not robots), whose actions can consciously or subconsciously lead to BIAS. "Any such trend or deviation from the truth in data collection, analysis, interpretation and publication is called bias" (Simundić, 2013). Let's think about where bias could have crept into the previous scenario (basically at all the points that humans are involved):

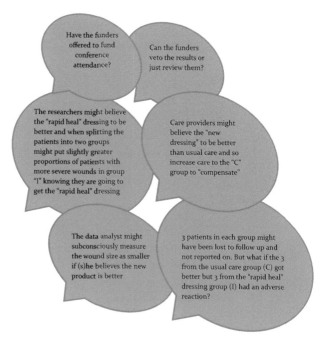

Figure 5.3 Bias "bubbles" – to show where bias could have crept in

Ok – so this is exaggerated – but I am trying to get you to appreciate that even with a design considered to be objective – and the best for establishing what works best – steps have to be built in to minimise bias because basically humans can consciously or subconsciously sway the results, making them less trustworthy. Do you remember in the previous chapter we mentioned post-positivists recognise it is impossible to be completely objective and try to minimise bias?

Now that you have some understanding of the basic logic underpinning the RCT design – that is, to manipulate one variable to see its effect on another variable whilst controlling other intrinsic or extrinsic variables through random allocation to groups and constancy of conditions, respectively (Bhide et al, 2018, Higgins et al, 2011, Jadad et al, 1996, Moher et al, 2010, Polit & Beck, 2018, Torgerson & Torgerson, 2008) – I would like to tell you about other RCT features that help to minimise bias (Higgins et al, 2011, Moher et al, 2010). To reiterate, these are necessary because humans can subconsciously, as well as consciously, do things that lead to bias.

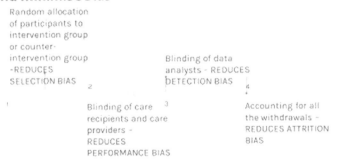

RCT features that improve design and minimise bias

Random allocation of participants to intervention group or counter-intervention group -REDUCES SELECTION BIAS

Blinding of data analysts - REDUCES DETECTION BIAS

Blinding of care recipients and care providers - REDUCES PERFORMANCE BIAS

Accounting for all the withdrawals - REDUCES ATTRITION BIAS

Figure 5.4 RCT features that improve design and minimise bias

Look again at Figure 5.4 (Higgins et al, 2011, Jadad et al, 1996, Schulz & Grimes, 2002) – what might the authors of our hypothetical trial be able to do to minimise the different types of bias?

> ## Box 5.2   Steps that could be taken to minimise bias in scenario 1
>
> True random allocation using a random number table, for example, and concealing this allocation until the point of allocation, for example, in a sealed opaque envelope to "rapid heal" dressing or alternative by a third party would prevent any influence by the researcher of how people were allocated to groups, thus **reducing selection bias.**
>
> If ethically possible, blinding care recipients (e.g. patients) and care providers (e.g. nurses) to whether patients had "rapid heal" dressing or alternative dressing would reduce performance bias (people acting differently when they know they are being observed) – but in truth this would have been difficult if the new dressing looked and felt different from the alternative product. So the study would **possibly be at risk of performance bias** – although less of a risk with a physiological outcome measure such as wound healing rather than subjective self-reporting.
>
> The person (e.g. the tissue viability nurse) assessing and analysing wound healing would not have needed to know who had received "rapid heal" dressing or the alternative if someone else had removed the dressings prior to assessment so she or he could assess the wounds essentially blinded – this would **reduce detection bias.**
>
> Explaining and accounting for why any patients had dropped out with reasons would help **reduce attrition bias.**
>
> I hope you can see you are starting to think critically about the research design.

It is also important to be aware of reporting bias – selective revealing or suppression of information (Stewart et al, 1996). This includes publication bias (studies that show a difference between interventions are published and cited more frequently than studies that don't show a difference – it doesn't necessarily mean they are better studies methodologically, but it might sell more journals). This means that we don't have the full picture. Selective reporting of results within a study can be another problem e.g. just reporting on the comfort of the dressing rather than its healing abilities, if the dressing performed better in relation to comfort, even though the original main aim was to look at its effect on healing. This means we come away with positive information about its comfort, potentially obscuring the information on its healing abilities.

Now instead of the effect of "rapid heal" dressing on chronic wounds in patients over 65, look at the "What works best" questions posed earlier from the different nursing fields. Use Table 5.1 and Figure 5.2 that I used to illustrate the hypothetical "rapid heal" dressing trial to help you set up hypothetical trials. Think about what would be ethical for the comparison "C" group to receive. Think about which intrinsic and extrinsic variables and sources of bias could affect the outcome and how you would try to control for these (tip: random allocation, constancy of conditions, blinding where possible). Think about how the outcome could be measured using a valid and reliable instrument.

Table 5.2 Examples of "what works best" questions from the four nursing fields

Adult field example: Does **topical negative pressure** heal chronic wounds?	Child field example: Does **emollient cream** resolve childhood eczema?
Mental health field example: Do **coping strategies** reduce stress in carers of relatives with dementia?	Learning disabilities field example: Does **exercise** reduce anxiety in people with a learning disability?

Table 5.3 ACP "what works best" question

ACP question:
In adults with radiation-induced oral mucositis, what is the effect of honey compared to 0.9% saline rinse on the presence or absence of oral mucositis and pain score?
Use Table 5.1 and Figures 5.2, 5.3, and 5.4 to design an ethical trial for this "what works best" research question. Have a go before looking.

Table 5.4 Basic steps in an RCT APPLIED TO THE HYPOTHETICAL SCENARIO$_2$

Remember I said earlier that with quantitative studies such as RCTs, it was about testing hypotheses. So the researcher proposes an RH, which wants to support a hunch. Often implicit is an NH, which seeks to nullify the hunch (Henkel, 1976, p. 36).	RH: If adults with radiation-induced oral mucositis are given medical-grade honey, then the presence of oral mucositis and pain score will be different from those given a standard treatment of 0.9% saline. (Note that I have said different rather than better; ethically, one should only conduct an RCT if there is **uncertainty** over what works best – honey could make outcomes worse.) NH: If adults with radiation-induced oral mucositis are given medical-grade honey, then the presence of oral mucositis and pain score will not be different from those given standard treatment of saline, and any observed difference will be due to chance.
Decide the intervention (I) and the counter-intervention (C)	I: medical-grade honey rinse C: 0.9% saline
Determine how the effect of I or C on the outcome (O) will be measured	Measure presence or absence of oral mucositis and pain scores at 1 week.
Identify the target population and select a random sample from it (P)	After obtaining ethical approval (which includes stopping guidance) to carry out the trial at several sites and hospitals that have adults being treated with radiation – randomly select 200 patients to try to obtain a representative sample. Explain the purpose of the study, its benefits, any risks, and the voluntary nature of taking part before obtaining their written informed consent. Take some baseline measurements.

(*Continued*)

Table 5.4 (Continued)

Randomly allocate half the sample to I and half to C	Leave it to chance how patients of varying age, gender, and illness severity are allocated to the two groups – to create two groups each containing 100 patients that are hopefully balanced for such variables (remember these are INTRINSIC variables).
Try to ensure constancy of conditions for both I and C	Give the same care as far as possible such as diet and pain medications to both groups of participants so they are treated the same apart from whether they receive I or C for oral mucositis (remember these are EXTRINSIC variables).
Collate scores	Measure in both groups of patients: 1. The presence or absence of oral mucositis at 1 week 2. The average pain score after 1 week
Analyse scores	Compare groups using an appropriate statistical approach – if using hypothesis testing and p values (Wilkinson, 2013): If p ≤ 0.05, it means the probability of getting the observed difference if chance was the only process operating (Gates, 2016) is very small ($<5\%$), so we reject the NH. If p >0.05, it means the probability of getting the observed difference if chance was the only process operating (Gates, 2016) is more than 5% – that's considered too big so unable to reject the NH.
Say if we can reject the NH or if we are unable to reject the NH (Campbell & Stanley, 1963, Wilkinson, 2013)	If we can reject the NH, the findings are said to be statistically significant. If we are unable to reject the NH, the findings are said to be not statistically significant.

Or if you prefer to see it represented as a picture "P" being the population of people with radiation-induced oral mucositis, with "I" being the honey, "C" being saline, and "O" being having/not having oral mucositis at week 1 and the pain scale score at week 1:

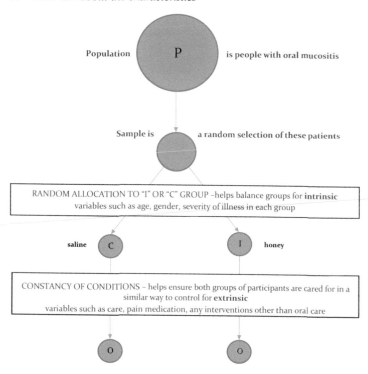

Figure 5.5 "Honey" RCT representation

Outcome 1: How many people have oral mucositis
after 1 week
Outcome 2: The average pain score after 1 week

Let's imagine that when outcomes (O) are compared, the group that received honey ("I") had lower rates of mucositis after 1 week compared to the saline group ("C") and the statistical test said p <0.05, meaning the probability of getting such a difference if chance was the only process operating is very small (less than 5%), so you could reject the NH and say this was a statistically significant finding. You might be tempted to conclude that the honey intervention "works best", right? Again, not necessarily . . .

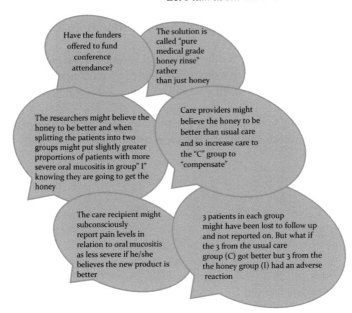

The solution is called "pure medical grade honey rinse" rather than just honey

Have the funders offered to fund conference attendance?

The researchers might believe the honey to be better and when splitting the patients into two groups might put slightly greater proportions of patients with more severe oral mucositis in group" I" knowing they are going to get the honey

Care providers might believe the honey to be better than usual care and so increase care to the "C" group to "compensate"

The care recipient might subconsciously report pain levels in relation to oral mucositis as less severe if he/she believes the new product is better

3 patients in each group might have been lost to follow up and not reported on. But what if the 3 from the usual care group (C) got better but 3 from the the honey group (I) had an adverse reaction

Figure 5.6 Bias "bubbles" – to show where bias could have crept in

Look again at Figure 5.4 indicating how to improve design and minimise bias – what might you be able to do to minimise the different types of bias if you were designing such a trial?

Box 5.3   Steps that could be taken to minimise bias in scenario 2

True random allocation using, for example, a random number table and concealing this allocation until the point of allocation in a sealed opaque envelope to honey or saline, for example, by a third party would prevent any influence by the researcher of how people were allocated to groups, thus **reducing selection bias.**

If ethically possible, blinding care recipients and care providers to whether patients had received honey or saline would reduce performance bias, but in truth this would have been difficult since honey and saline look, feel, and taste different. So the study would **possibly be at risk of performance bias** – if people believe they are having a new treatment, they might report less pain, for example, one of the outcomes.

The person looking for the presence or absence of oral mucositis would not have needed to know who had received honey or saline so she or he could assess it essentially blinded – this would **reduce detection bias**.

Explaining and accounting for why any patients had dropped out with reasons would help **reduce attrition bias**.

Summary

- An RCT is a research approach designed to answer a **"what works best"** question to try to see if there is a cause and effect relationship.
- It is often described as an objective approach and is the top primary research design in the quantitative hierarchy of evidence, although post-positivists recognise that human beings carry out RCTs and need to take steps to minimise bias.
- It is the **ONLY** research design that features RANDOM ALLOCATION to groups, which helps to control for intrinsic variables and therefore minimises selection bias.
- The same care or constancy of conditions is desirable where possible for both groups to help control for extrinsic variables.
- From a design point of view, blinding of care providers and care recipients to reduce performance bias, blinding of data analysts to reduce detection bias, and accounting for any withdrawals (with reasons) to reduce attrition bias are also deemed desirable by methodologists. This is not always possible, of course.
- RCT researchers should report on all outcomes to reduce selective reporting bias.
- Ethical approval and informed consent are vital for RCTs to ensure, for example, that comparison groups receive current EBP and that ongoing data analysis and stopping guidance are built into the RCT protocol so if one treatment outperforms the other, all can benefit from effective intervention (Moher et al, 2010). Participants should also know they have the right to remain anonymous, refuse to participate, or withdraw at any time without it affecting care.

- Before any results can be trusted, the RCT design needs to be examined closely to see if it has been conducted appropriately.
- Appreciating this is further developing your critical appraisal skills.

References

Bhide A, Shah PS, Acharya G. (2018) A simplified guide to randomized controlled trials. *Acta Obstetricia et Gynecologica Scandinavica*; 97(4): 380–387. doi: 10.1111/aogs.13309.

Campbell DT, Stanley JC. (1963) *Experimental and Quasi-experimental Designs for Research*. Chicago: Rand McNally & Company.

Gates S. Blog. (2016) *The Probability That the Results Are Due to Chance*. 12/11/2016, Evidence-based everything (warwick.ac.uk)

Henkel RE. (1976) *Tests of Significance*. Newbury Park, London and New Delhi: Sage publications.

Higgins JPT, Altman DG, Gotzsche PC, Juni P, Moher D, Oxman AD. et al. (2011) The Cochrane collaboration's tool for assessing risk of bias in randomised trials. *BMJ*; 343: d5928. doi: 10.1136/bmj.d5928

Jadad AR, Moore RA, Carroll D, Jenkinson C, Reynolds DJM., Gavaghan DJ, Mcquay HJ. (1996) Assessing the quality of reports of randomized clinical trials: Is blinding necessary? *Controlled Clinical Trials*; 17(1): 1–12.

Moher D, Hopewell S, Schulz KF, Montori V, Gøtzsche PC, Devereaux PJ, Elbourne D, Egger M, Altman DG. (2010) CONSORT 2010 explanation and elaboration: updated guidelines for reporting parallel group randomised trials. *BMJ; 340*: c869.

Polit DF, Beck CT. (2018) *Essentials of Nursing Research: Appraising Evidence for Nursing Practice*. 9th edn. Philadelphia. Wolters Kluwer.

Schulz KF, Grimes DA. (2002) Generation of allocation sequences in randomised trials: Chance, not choice. *Lancet*; 359(9305): 515–519.

Simundić AM. (2013) Bias in research. *Biochemia Medica*; 23(1): 12–15. doi: 10.11613/bm.2013.003

Stewart LA, Parmar MK. (1996) Bias in the analysis and reporting of randomized controlled trials. *International Journal of Technology Assessment in Health Care; 12*(2): 264–275.

Torgerson DJ, Torgerson CJ. (2008) *Designing Randomised Trials in Health, Education and the Social Sciences*. Houndmills, Basingstoke, Hampshire: Palgrave Macmillan.

US National Library of Medicine. (2008) *RCT Definition*.

Wilkinson M. (2013) Testing the null hypothesis: the forgotten legacy of Karl Popper? *Journal of Sports Science; 31*(9): 919–920. doi: 10.1080/02640414.2012.753636. Epub 2012 December 19. PMID: 2324

6 Some non-randomised quantitative designs – quasi-experiments, cohort studies, and case-control studies

The previous chapter discussed the RCT quantitative design, which tries to establish if the variable X – "rapid heal" – caused variable Y – wound healing. Other authors might refer to the intervention (I) causing the outcome (O) – (remember PICO)?

It is worth spending some time considering the criteria for inferring causal relationships by John Stuart Mills (Polit & Beck, 2018, p. 139) because it will help you appreciate why RCTs are the top primary quantitative design for establishing the effectiveness of interventions and why the quantitative designs considered in this chapter sit below it.

1. A cause must precede an effect in time. This means you must ascertain that the application of "rapid heal" happened before the chronic wound healing occurred.
2. There must be an empirical relationship between the presumed cause and the presumed effect. This means that a greater number of wounds were observed to have healed in the "rapid heal" group compared to the control/comparison group.
3. The relationship cannot be explained as being the result of the influence of other extraneous variables. This means that the improved healing can't be due to anything other than the "rapid heal". It is this last criteria that presents the most problems for researchers, especially with non-randomised, less controlled studies.

An RCT does the most relatively, in design terms, to try to rule out "other/extraneous variables", which as you saw in the previous chapter

DOI: 10.4324/9781003156017-9

could be intrinsic (things within the individual that might affect the outcome) or extrinsic (things external to the individual that might affect the outcome). A well-designed RCT also takes steps to minimise conscious or subconscious bias from humans. Another way of putting it is it does the most to try to rule out alternative explanations.

It is generally accepted by quantitative researchers that random allocation (done truly randomly and concealed prior to implementation) of a large sample of people leaves it to chance that variations in known intrinsic variables (things within the individual that may affect the outcome like nutritional status, weight, overall health, grade of wound – even things we don't know about) would be distributed evenly in both groups. A silly example would be hair colour. Random allocation would also leave it to chance that variations in hair colour would be distributed evenly in both groups.

So a balancing of known and unknown variables is achievable, albeit not guaranteed, with random allocation of a large sample of people. Another way of putting it is it helps prevent systematic differences between the two groups (selection bias) of baseline characteristics (Odgaard-Jensen et al, 2011). If it is left to chance, the researcher can't select who goes into which group. **This is the great strength of RCTs** – although it is always worth checking the equivalence of the two groups when you read a published trial (it is usually the first table) to see if random allocation achieved this equivalence/balancing of (intrinsic) baseline characteristics.

This gives us more confidence that if the sample size is large and the two groups are balanced like this to minimise selection bias, and there is constancy of conditions (as much as there can be in real-world enquires) for both groups (to control for extrinsic variables like turning schedules, diet provided in hospital setting) and steps have been taken to minimise other sources of bias (such as performance, detection, attrition, and reporting), when we compare the "rapid heal" to the alternative product, we are more likely to obtain an unbiased estimate of what is going on.

If all this randomisation and control are necessary to try to show cause and effect – if such a relationship exists between two variables – why then do we have quasi-experiments, cohort, and case-control designs?

Sometimes it is either practically, technically, or ethically impossible to randomly allocate to an "I" or "C" group but the researcher is still interested in the relationship between variables to try to understand what is going on in order to try to provide the best care. Let me give you some examples to show you what I mean:

What is the effect of a fluid, fibre, and exercise programme on the bowel function of a group of residents in a care home?

You might want to evaluate if something new such as an "increased fluid, fibre, and exercise" programme works, but how can you if it is to be introduced to all the residents in that care home?

What are the effects of eating disorders on bone mineral density?

Is it technically possible to randomly allocate to having an eating disorder or not? Of course not!

What are the effects of passive smoking on children's health?

Is it ethically feasible to randomly allocate children to growing up with parents that smoke or not? Of course not!

This doesn't stop you from being interested in the relationship between these variables in order to provide the best care, but to understand these "I" effects (if any), there are other **non-randomised** quantitative designs such as quasi-experiments, cohort studies, and case-control studies that explore them – and these are the focus of this chapter.

In these **non-randomised studies (NRSs)**, from a research design point of view, the lack of random assignment to groups means this balancing of known and unknown intrinsic variables is lost. And even with the use of methods to address other sources of bias, such studies are still at risk of selection bias, and people might wrongly conclude an intervention or exposure to something is having an effect when it was in fact due to another variable (Gerstein et al, 2019, Rush et al, 2018).

So these studies can only try to look for association rather than causation – and as such appear lower in the quantitative hierarchy of evidence than SRs of RCTs or RCTs themselves.

So rather than looking to see if X causes Y, or "I" causes "O", they look to see if X is ASSOCIATED with Y (or "I" is associated with "O").

Box 6.1   Quasi-experiments: description

- Consider the research question "what is the effect of a fluid, fibre, and exercise programme on the bowel function of a group of care home residents?" Remember we can still use the research process as a guide:

1. The researchers are seeking to explore the effectiveness of an intervention to test a hypothesis or to evaluate an intervention.

    ▼

2. A **quasi-experimental** approach is characterized by **no random assignment** of participants to the experimental or control/comparison group, but **there is still manipulation of the independent variable/intervention** (Campbell & Stanley, 1963): *Non-equivalent control group design* – one care home has the new programme, another similar care home doesn't, and measurement of the dependent variable/outcome – average number of bowel movements at each home – is compared. *Non-interrupted time series design* – one care home has the new programme (i.e. increased fluid, fibre, and exercise), and there is no comparison home, but instead multiple measures of bowel movements are made before and after the introduction of the programme. A third, better quasi-experimental design would be a combination of these two designs. There would be some control over other/extraneous variables but not the intrinsic ones.

    ▼

3. Collect quantitative data in a way that is valid and reliable.

    ▼

4. Analyse the **quantitative** data.

    ▼

5. Disseminate the findings.

Here I am trying to show you that with an "is there an association" type question the researchers may use a quasi-experiment in order to research it and how a quasi-experiment follows the research process. From this brief overview you can see it has certain characteristics and is still a quantitative research approach, but it differs from the RCT in that although it is prospective (looks forward in time) and involves manipulation of the independent variable/intervention, it **lacks random allocation** to groups. For this reason it is difficult to know how similar the two groups being compared are apart from one group having the fluid, fibre, and exercise programme.

Think about what you know about RCTs and what type of bias a quasi-experiment could be at risk of.

Box 6.2   Cohort studies: description

- Consider again the research question "What are the effects of eating disorders on bone mineral density" and use the research process as a guide.

1. The researchers want to see whether in a defined group of people followed over time, there are associations between a particular intervention/exposure to something and a particular outcome (Mann, 2003, Reeves et al, 2008).

    ▾

2. Using a cohort approach, they would select a sample of participants. Some of these participants will have been exposed to the factor(s) of interest, and some of these participants will not have been exposed (or to a lesser degree).

    ▾

3. They would follow up with the participants. Some of the participants who develop the disease, illness, or symptoms being investigated (in this example, osteoporosis) will have been exposed to the factor of interest (in this example, having an eating disorder). Some will not have been exposed (or less exposed). These studies often involve thousands of participants over many years.

    ▾

4. They would analyse results **to see if the risk of developing the disease, illness, or symptom (in this example, osteoporosis) is greater in one of the two groups.**

    ▾

5. They would disseminate the findings.

Here I am trying to show you that an "is there an association" type question can use a cohort study to research it and how a cohort study follows the research process. You can see it has certain characteristics and is still a quantitative research approach, but it differs from the RCT in that although it is prospective (looks forward in time), it **lacks manipulation of the intervention/ exposure** – this is naturally occurring, and as such, **it lacks random allocation** to groups, so it is difficult to know how similar the two groups being compared are at baseline apart from one group having the exposure (an eating disorder). Some matching might be possible, but you could only match for known variables such as age and geographical location. Following is a visual representation of if there appeared to be an association – the difficulty is other variables could be associated with the outcome too. It would certainly warrant further investigation though.

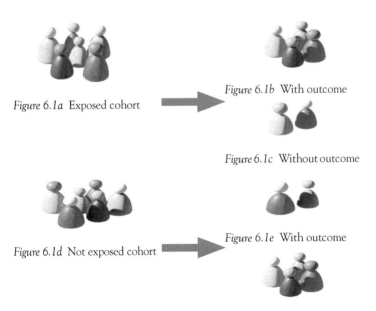

Figure 6.1a Exposed cohort

Figure 6.1b With outcome

Figure 6.1c Without outcome

Figure 6.1d Not exposed cohort

Figure 6.1e With outcome

Figure 6.1f Without outcome

Box 6.3   Case-control studies: description

- Consider again the research question "What are the effects of passive smoking on children's health?" and use the research process as a guide:

1. In this type of study the researchers compare people with a specific outcome of interest (cases) with "people from the same source population but without that outcome (controls) to examine the association between the outcome and prior exposure (or intervention)" (Mann, 2003, Reeves et al, 2008).

   ▼

2. Using a case-control approach, the researchers would need an identification of cases – the children with the disease or outcome and an identification of controls – that is, the children who do not have the disease or outcome but are similar in age, with similar histories and environment.

   ▼

3. There would be measurement of the factor of interest (in this example, passive smoking), as well as other potentially confounding factors.

   ▼

4. There would be analysis of whether or not the cases (in this example, children with poorer lung health, e.g. asthma) were more likely than the controls (children with good lung health) to have been exposed to a risk factor (in this example, passive smoking). Results are analysed **to see if the odds of being exposed to a risk factor (in this case, passive smoking) is greater in one of the two groups.**

   ▼

5. There would be dissemination of the findings.

Here I am trying to show you that an "is there an association" type question can use a case-control study to research it and how this follows the research process. From this brief overview, you can see it has certain characteristics and is still a quantitative research approach, but it differs from the RCT in that it is **retrospective** (looks back in time). As the exposure/intervention and outcome will already have occurred, it obviously **lacks manipulation** and **lacks random allocation**, and there would be **less opportunity for control** by gathering information retrospectively, so it is difficult to know how similar the two groups being compared are apart from one group having the outcome (e.g. asthma). Even if the researcher tries to match cases with controls regarding age and similar histories, **what other variables might they have been exposed to?**

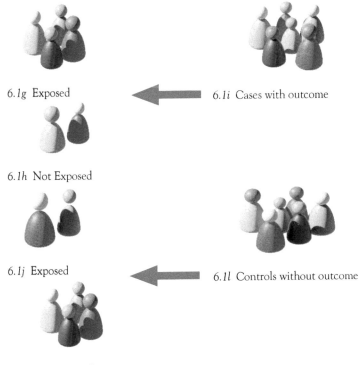

6.1g Exposed

6.1i Cases with outcome

6.1h Not Exposed

6.1j Exposed

6.1l Controls without outcome

6.1k Not Exposed

Cohort studies and case-control studies are used a lot in epidemiology, which studies how often diseases occur in different groups of people and why. Now look at the "is there an association" questions **posed earlier** from the different nursing fields. Use Boxes 6.1, 6.2, and 6.3 to help you set up hypothetical, non-randomised quantitative studies.

Table 6.1 Examples of "is there an association with" question from the different nursing fields

Adult field example: Is there an association between vaping and lung disease?	Child field example: Done
Mental health field example: Done	Learning disabilities field example: Is there an association between socioeconomic background and accessing support services?

Table 6.2 The SIDS example as a potential case-control study

HV question:

In infants under 1, is there an association between soft bedding and sudden infant death syndrome (SIDS) cases?

Answer:

P	Infants
I	Soft bedding
C	Non-soft bedding
O	Rates of SIDS
D	This is an "is there an association" type question, usually referring to cohort studies or case-control studies to explore it

Sample search strategy answer:

P	I	C	O	D
#1 Bab* **OR** Infant* **OR** Under 1 year old **OR** Newborn	#2 Soft bedding **OR** Soft blanket **OR** Duvet **OR** Quilt **OR** Pillow	Non-soft bedding	#3 Sudden infant death rates **OR** SIDS rates **OR** Cot death rates	Cohort **OR** Case-control studies

#1 **AND** #2 **AND** #3 would provide a specific basic search strategy for evidence on soft baby sleeping products (and any other names for it) for infants under 1 (and any other terms for babies) from appropriate quantitative research designs that consider is there an association with/or looking back, was there an association with bedding type and SIDS rates.

Box 6.4   Hypothetical case-control study exploring SIDS

- Consider the research question "in infants under 1 is there an association between the type of sleep covering and sudden infant death syndrome (SIDS) cases" and use the research process as a guide:

1. This research might be of interest if you were a health visitor and you were asked by parents about the guidance about which bedding can be safely used for their babies. The researchers might have wanted to find out in the babies who sadly died from SIDS if there was an "exposure" to a factor that was different from babies that didn't. In this example, it would have compared babies with a specific outcome of interest (cases) with babies from the same source population but without that outcome (controls) to see if there was an association between the outcome (SIDS) and prior exposure (e.g. having a particular bedding type).

2. The researchers may have used a case-control approach and identified cases – the babies with the disease or outcome (SIDS) – and controls – the babies who did not have the disease or outcome (no SIDS).

3. They would have measured the factor of interest (in this example, the type of bedding), as well as other potentially confounding factors.

4. There would have been analysis of whether or not the cases were more likely than the controls to have been exposed to a risk factor. Results would be analysed to see if the odds of being exposed to a potential risk factor (in this case, a particular bedding type) was greater in one of the two groups.

5. There would be dissemination of the findings.

Here I am trying to show you that for an "is there an association" type question researchers may use a case-control study to research it and how this follows the research process. From this brief overview you can see it has certain characteristics and is still a quantitative research approach, but it differs from the RCT in that it is **retrospective** (looks back in time). As the exposure and outcome will already have occurred, it obviously **lacks manipulation** and **lacks random allocation**, and there would be **less control** when gathering information retrospectively. So it would be difficult to know how similar the two groups being compared were apart from one of the groups of babies having SIDS. Even if the researcher tried to match cases with controls regarding their age, birth weight, and similar histories, there may have been other variables they have been exposed to in the past.

Non-randomised studies look for association rather than causation. Other variables may also associated with the outcome – not just the one being studied. In common with RCTs, in quasi- experiments, cohort, and case-control studies (all referred to as NRSs by Cochrane) dimensions of bias that include selection, performance, detection, attrition, and reporting bias should still be considered (Reeves et al, 2008). Cohort studies can resolve the time order of events and examine study outcomes over a longer time period but are at risk of selection bias and attrition bias due to the lengths of these studies. Case-control studies are useful when an outcome takes a long time to develop or is rare, but are at risk of selection bias, recall bias, and multifactorial causes (Polit & Beck, 2018, Reeves et al, 2008).

Summary

- Quantitative researchers are often very interested in the relationship between variables in order to understand what is going on in order to be able to provide the best care.
- Although the great strength of random allocation from a design point of view is the balancing of groups for known and unknown intrinsic variables, sometimes it is either practically, technically, or ethically impossible to do this.

- A good appreciation of RCT design features, however (**random allocation to groups, manipulation, and control**), helps you to understand what is missing in design terms from quasi-experiment and observational studies such as cohort and case-control studies and why they have to **build in other steps** to help minimise sources of bias.
- The non-randomised studies are all still at risk of selection bias (individual differences in the two groups being compared), as not all known and unknown intrinsic variables can have been balanced.
- These studies will also have had less control over extrinsic variables because in naturally occurring situations, one can't have constancy of conditions.
- A quasi-experiment is a **prospective** quantitative research approach.
- It sits below the RCT in the quantitative hierarchy of evidence because even though the intervention is still given to one group (so it **has manipulation**), it **lacks random allocation** to groups because it is practically not feasible to do so.
- A cohort study is a **prospective** research approach designed to see if exposure to "X" results in a greater incidence of "Y" (Reeves et al, 2008).
- It sits below the quasi-experiment in the quantitative hierarchy of evidence, as it **lacks manipulation** of the intervention/exposure and **lacks random allocation** to groups because it is usually ethically or technically not feasible to do so and the intervention/exposure occurs naturally.
- A case-control study is a **retrospective** research approach that looks back in time to see if a greater prevalence of "Y" was as a result of exposure to "X" (Reeves et al, 2008).
- It sits below the cohort design in the quantitative hierarchy of evidence – as the intervention/exposure and outcome will already have occurred naturally – thus it obviously **lacks manipulation** of the exposure, **lacks random allocation**, and **there would be less opportunity for control by** gathering information retrospectively.
- No study can prove causation 100%, but there is a spectrum of quantitative designs that try to explain and explore the

relationships between variables, with RCT above quasi-experiments, which is above cohort, which is above case-control designs – as more is built into the design to control for intrinsic and extrinsic variables and to minimise systematic variation (bias), the higher up the hierarchy of evidence you go.

* This means the higher up the hierarchy you go, the higher the internal validity of the study (its ability to show X causes Y, or I causes O).

* Appreciating this is further developing your critical appraisal skills of quantitative research designs.

References

Campbell DT, Stanley JC. (1963) *Experimental and Quasi-experimental Designs for Research*. Chicago: Rand McNally & Company.

Gerstein HC, McMurray J, Holman RR. (2019) Real-world studies no substitute for RCTs in establishing efficacy. *Lancet*; 393: 210–211.

Mann CJ. (2003) Observational research methods. Research design II: cohort, cross sectional, and case-control studies. *Emergency Medicine Journal*; 20(1): 54–60.

Odgaard-Jensen J, Vist GE, Timmer A, Kunz R, Akl EA, Schünemann H, Briel M, Nordmann AJ, Pregno S, Oxman AD. (2011) Randomisation to protect against selection bias in healthcare trials. *Cochrane Database System Review*; 2011(4) April 13: MR000012. doi: 10.1002/14651858.MR000012. pub3. PMID: 21491415; PMCID: PMC7150228.

Polit DF, Beck CT. (2018) *Essentials of Nursing Research: Appraising Evidence for Nursing Practice*. 9th edn. Philadelphia. Wolters Kluwer.

Reeves BC, Deeks JJ, Higgins JPT, Wells GA. (2008) Chapter 13: Including non-randomised studies. In Higgins JPT, Green S (Eds) *Cochrane Handbook of Systematic Reviews of Interventions*. Chichester: John Wiley & Sons.

Rush CJ, Campbell RT, Jhund PS, Petrie MC, McMurray JJV. (2018) Association is not causation: Treatment effects cannot be estimated from observational data in heart failure. *European Heart Journal*; 39: 3417–3438.

7 What are effect measures for dichotomous outcomes?

Ok – it has probably felt a bit intense the last few chapters as I talked you through some quantitative randomised and non-randomised designs, and we haven't even gotten to how to critically appraise quantitative research fully yet!

This is because as well as being able to judge if research designs are ethical and trustworthy, you also need to understand if how the data has been **collected** and **analysed** is APPROPRIATE and you can INTERPRET the results, and it is this we will focus on in the next two chapters.

Let's consider once again the "what works best" question for the fictitious product "rapid heal" on chronic wounds. Imagine you have found a pertinent RCT whilst searching the literature, and as you are reading it you can see it follows the research process, and you are noticing the steps the authors have taken to control for variables and to minimise bias. This is great and consolidating your learning so far.

Table 7.1 Hypothetical trial looking at fictitious "rapid heal" on chronic wounds summary

1. The conceptual phase	In the background of your article, the burden and current management of chronic wounds have been discussed and the possibility that "rapid heal" may have a positive effect on healing.

(Continued)

DOI: 10.4324/9781003156017-10

Table 7.1 (Continued)

2. The design and planning phase	The authors have set up the hypotheses, and they have chosen an RCT to try to test them. After gaining ethical approval, they have randomly selected, then randomly allocated, 200 consenting patients over 65 with a chronic wound to either "rapid heal" or the best alternative dressing currently used for chronic wounds. The nursing team have been briefed to provide the same diet and turning schedules to improve constancy of conditions. Steps have been taken to minimise bias where possible.
3. The empirical or data collection phase	The wounds have been assessed by the same tissue viability nurse (TVN), who was blind to who had received which dressing. The TVN looked to see: 1. How many wounds have not healed or healed in each group after 6 weeks 2. The average reduction in wound surface area in each group after 2 weeks
4. The analytic phase.	The authors presented the results as: 1. Wounds remaining **unhealed** at 6 weeks as a **risk ratio** of 0.8 with a 95% confidence interval of 0.4 to 1.2 2. The average **reduction** in wound surface area at 2 weeks as a **mean difference** of 1.3 cm² with a 95% confidence interval of –0.1 cm² to 2.7 cm² Don't worry if you don't understand these terms yet – we will go over them in this and the next chapter – these are the **effect measures**.
5. The dissemination phase	

If you prefer to see it represented as a picture, with "P" being the population of people over 65 with a chronic wound, "I" being the fictitious "rapid heal" dressing, "C" being the current evidence-based dressing recommended for a chronic wound, and "O" being the number of chronic wounds remaining unhealed after 6 weeks and the mean reduction in wound surface area after 2 weeks, see the following figure.

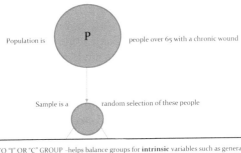

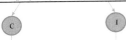

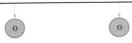

Figure 7.1 "Rapid heal" RCT representation

Data analyst is blinded to reduce detection bias. All patients are followed up to reduce attrition bias.

1. **In relation to wounds remaining unhealed at 6 weeks, the authors have presented <u>a risk ratio of 0.8 with a 95% confidence interval of 0.4 to 1.2.</u>**

2. **In relation to the average reduction in wound surface area at 2 weeks, they have presented this as a <u>mean difference of 1.3 cm^2 with a 95% confidence interval of −0.1 cm^2 to 2.7 cm^2.</u>**

As I said earlier don't worry if you don't understand these terms yet. These are the **effect measures** – we will go over them in this and the next chapter.

I would like to go over a couple of things with you before we discuss **effect measures**. If you are feeling brave, read the next several paragraphs. If not, go straight to Box 7.1 and recommence reading there. When a trial is carried out on a random **sample**, researchers want to be able to make inferences (draw conclusions) about what is found out to the target **population**, i.e. to generalise. Two inferential methods are available to do this – (null) **hypothesis testing using p values** and **estimation using confidence intervals** (Freeman & Julious, 2021). Because you will come across both when reading research, I would like to provide brief descriptions of each so that, even if you don't have an in-depth knowledge of statistics, you will still be able to make some sense of these values. I have found that students are much more motivated to learn about EBP if they can interpret figures that previously they struggled to understand.

Hypothesis testing using p values

In Chapter 5 when talking about RCTs, I briefly alluded to hypothesis testing using p values. With this inferential method, the researcher usually starts with a hunch that an intervention will have an effect on an outcome and formulates a research hypothesis (RH). A null hypothesis (NH) starts with the "gloomy" position that there is nothing new happening or assumes the experiment will not work (Clegg, 1990) or that any observed difference is due to chance. Understandably, a lot of students think it is the RH being tested with statistical tests, but it is actually the NH (Wilkinson, 2013). Let me try to explain that a bit . . .

Probability-based statistics "looks" at the obtained result/**difference** and asks "What is the likelihood/probability of seeing a result/difference of that size/magnitude that you are seeing in your sample in the population IF IT WAS JUST CHANCE OPERATING?"

A high probability (by convention, p >0.05) tells us we <u>are likely</u> to see a difference of that size if only chance is operating (Gates, 2016) – so we **can't reject the NH**. The result is deemed to be *not statistically significant*.

A low probability (by convention, p ≤0.05) tells us we <u>are unlikely</u> to see a difference of that size if only chance is operating (Gates, 2016), so we **reject the NH**. The result is deemed to be *statistically significant*.

So you see, the RH hypothesis cannot be tested directly; "it is accepted by exclusion if the test of statistical significance rejects the null hypothesis" (Banerjee et al, 2009).

This is how I make sense of it for myself in relation to our "rapid heal" example:

- *An RH (says there is a relationship between the "rapid heal" and the healing).*
- *And an NH (which says there is no relationship or no effect exists).*
- *You carry out the experiment/RCT on your **sample** – you get a result/**difference** which shows more wounds have healed with "rapid heal" than with the alternative dressing – say, 20% more.*
- *Statistical evaluation "looks" at that result/difference in relation to the NH – could you get a difference of the size you are seeing in your sample (e.g. 20%) in the **population** JUST BY CHANCE ALONE (Breakwell et al, 1995, p. 347)?*
- *So if you see **p >0.05,** it means it's likely that you could just see this difference of 20% due to chance; therefore, you **can't reject the null**/chance explanation – you might conclude from this **one sample** that the "rapid heal" didn't work and the prediction has failed (read Popper if you want to understand falsification [Wilkinson, 2013]).*
- *But if you see **p ≤0.05,** it indicates you probably couldn't get this difference of 20% just due to chance (well, only 5% or less of the time anyway); therefore, you **can reject the null**/chance explanation – the researcher might conclude "rapid heal" has worked.*
- ***This means 5% of the time we could draw the wrong conclusion** – this is why we can't say we have proved a hypothesis, and this is why there is value in replication (essentially using lots of samples/RCTs).*

Estimation using confidence intervals

Some researchers argue that "this threshold was never developed to allow researchers or clinicians to make yes/no conclusions that, if a p-value is greater than 0.05, the intervention has no effect and, if a p-value is less than 0.05, the intervention has an effect" (McCormack, 2013).

When research is carried out, it is usually on only one (randomly selected) sample – not the total population – so an observed difference from one RCT is referred to as a *point estimate*.

With this second inferential method (where you still want to infer things about a sample to a target population), the researcher usually starts with a point estimate from a sample. Probability-based statistics can be used to calculate an *interval estimate* – also known as a confidence interval (CI) – **a range of values** – based on the sample data in which the population value for such a **difference** may lie (Gardner and Altman, 1986).

Devore (2008, chapter 7) describes the confidence level 95% as "not so much a statement about any particular interval. Instead it pertains to what would happen if a very large number of like intervals were to be constructed using the same CI formula". So if you had 100 intervals from a 100 samples, you would be confident that 95 of them would contain the population value.

So with this method a point estimate is usually accompanied by an interval estimate/CI. This helps indicate the precision of the estimate (du Prel et al, 2009), and conclusions about statistical significance are possible with the help of the CI.

If the 95% CI **includes the "no difference" value**, this would be considered **not a statistically significant result**.

If the 95% CI **doesn't include the "no difference" value**, this would be considered **a statistically significant result**.

This is how I make sense of it for myself:

- *You carry out the experiment/RCT on your **sample** – you get a result/**difference** – a point estimate e.g. 20% more healing with "rapid heal".*
- *Statistical evaluation involves calculating an interval estimate – so rather than one point estimate from a sample, there is **a range of values instead**, in which the population value for such a difference may lie.*
- *If the **95% CI contains the "no difference" value** – so in this example, a range of values from, say, 0% to 40% (with 0% difference being the no difference result here), because it indicates a range of plausible values for your population for 95% of the intervals, you **cannot be confident a difference exists** between "rapid heal" and the alternative.*
- *If the **95% CI does not contain the "no difference" value** – so in this example, a range of values from, say, 10% to 30%, because it indicates a range of plausible values for your population for 95% of*

*the intervals, you **can be more confident a difference exists** between the "rapid heal" and the alternative.*

- *This is equivalent to carrying out a hypothesis test (Sheldon, 2008, p. 86).*
- *Don't forget, though, that if you drew 100 samples at random, only 95% of the intervals would contain the population parameter. You only have one sample, so you **take the risk 5% of the time that you might not have the true result**. So again, there is value in replication (essentially using lots of samples/RCTs).*

"P-values enable the recognition of any statistically noteworthy findings whereas confidence intervals provides a range in which the true value lies with a certain degree of probability" (du Prel et al, 2009, p. 335), so they advocate reporting both. Estimation using CIs is not new, but adopting them widely is now more common (Cumming, 2014, Freeman & Julious, 2021). You will see these values a lot in systematic reviews. For that reason the next two chapters focus on **effect measures** for dichotomous and continuous outcomes and **estimation using CIs** in order to give you experience in interpreting them.

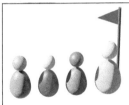

Figure 7.2 Follow me

Box 7.1   Dichotomous outcomes

This may mean very little to you at present, but bear with me – I am going to guide you through it so you can see:

a)   if the analysis is APPROPRIATE
       and
b)   if you can INTERPRET the results

So with our fictitious dressing "rapid heal", we are looking if it is having any effect on chronic wound healing vs. alternative dressing on the number of wounds healed or not healed at 6 weeks. Remember we hope to generalise these findings to a target population. For this we need **effect measures**, which are statistical constructs that compare outcome data between two groups. Effect measures can broadly be divided into **ratio** measures (dealt with in this chapter) and **difference** measures (dealt with in the next chapter) (Higgins & Deeks, 2021).

Risks and risk ratios

> **Box 7.2   Hypothetical trial looking at the effect of "rapid heal" on healing and not healing wounds**
>
> Let us consider first the number of wounds healed at 6 weeks. First of all you need to understand that this is a <u>dichotomous</u>/binary outcome – this just means you can be in one of two states at the end of the study period – in our example, either not healed or healed at 6 weeks.

One way of looking at this is to ask: what is your risk of not healing if you are in the experimental/I/"rapid heal" group? Let's call this R_E.

What is your risk of not healing if you are in the control/C/ alternative dressing group? Let's call this R_C.

So here we have two risks: R_E and R_C.

A way of comparing these two risks is to **divide** R_E by R_C – this is an <u>effect measure</u> and is called a **risk ratio or a relative risk** (by convention, the experimental risk is usually divided by the control risk) (Alderson & Green, 2002).

So let me show you a useful table:

Table 7.2 2 × 2 table

	Event: remaining unhealed at 6 weeks	Non-event: healing at 6 weeks	Total
Experimental group (I/"rapid heal" group)	20	80	100
Control group (C/alternative dressing)	25	75	100

$$R_E = \frac{\text{having the event (remaining unhealed at 6 weeks with "rapid heal")}}{\text{total}}$$

$$R_E = 20/100$$

$$R_C = \frac{\text{having the event (remaining unhealed at 6 weeks with alternative dressing)}}{\text{total}}$$

$R_C = 25/100$

To compare the two risks or likelihoods, we can calculate a risk ratio (RR):

$$RR = \frac{20/100}{25/100}$$

$$RR = 0.8$$

Whenever you see an RR, ask yourselves if the RR is less than 1 ($<$1), greater than 1 ($>$1), or equal to 1 ($=$ 1) and what does this tell us about Events happening in the Experimental group?

If the **RR was $<$1** it would tell us **events were happening LESS in the experimental group** (little number divided by a bigger number gives us a number less than 1, e.g. 5/100 divided by 25/100 gives us 0.2).

If the **RR was $>$1** it would tell us **events were happening MORE in the experimental group** (big number divided by a smaller number gives us a number greater than 1, e.g. 50/100 divided by 25/100 gives us 2).

If the **RR was $=$ 1** (or very close to 1) it would tell us **events were happening at the SAME rate in both groups** (any number divided by itself gives us 1, e.g. 25/100 divided by 25/100 gives us 1). This would indicate **NO DIFFERENCE** between the two groups/interventions.

Box 7.3   Interpretation of RR

In this case the **RR = 0.8, which is $<$1 and tells us Events (remaining unhealed at 6 weeks) are happening LESS in the experimental ("rapid heal") group** than in the control (C/ alternative dressing) group: little number (20/100) divided by a bigger number (25/100) gives us a number less than 1 – in this example 0.8.

Essentially your **risk/likelihood** of remaining unhealed at 6 weeks with this hypothetical data is essentially 0.8 times **less** with "rapid heal" when compared to the alternative dressing. "Rapid heal" reduced the risk to 80% of what it would have been. Thus, "rapid heal" reduced the risk by 20% of what it was in the control group.

Odds and odds ratios

Sometimes you might see results expressed as another <u>effect measure</u> called an **odds ratio** rather than a risk ratio, e.g. in a case-control study. They are interpreted in a similar way, although you would talk about odds rather than risks.

So what are your odds of remaining unhealed if you are in the experimental/I/"rapid heal" group? Let's call this O$_E$.

What are your odds of remaining unhealed if you are in the control/C/alternative dressing group? Let's call this O$_C$.

Here we have two odds: O$_E$ and O$_C$. A way of comparing the two odds is to **divide** O$_E$ by O$_C$ – this is called an **odds ratio** (Alderson & Green, 2002).

So referring to the same useful table:

Table 7.3 2 × 2 table

	Event: remaining unhealed at 6 weeks	Non-Event: healing at 6 weeks	Total
Experimental group (I/"rapid heal" group)	20	80	100
Control group (C/alternative dressing)	25	75	100

$$O_E = \frac{\text{having the event (remaining unhealed at 6 weeks with "rapid heal")}}{\text{Not having the event (healing at 6 weeks)}}$$

$$O_E = 20/80$$

$$O_C = \frac{\text{having the event (remaining unhealed at 6 weeks with alternative dressing)}}{\text{Not having the event (healing at 6 weeks)}}$$

$$O_C = 25/75$$

To compare the two odds, we can calculate an odds ratio:

$$OR = \frac{20/80}{25/75}$$

$$OR = 0.75$$

In this case the **OR = 0.75,** which is **less than 1** and that tells us **Events (remaining unhealed at 6 weeks) are happening less in the**

experimental ("rapid heal") group than in the control (C/alternative dressing) group (smaller number 20/80 divided by a bigger number 25/75 gives us a number less than 1). Essentially your **odds** of remaining unhealed with this hypothetical data is essentially **0.75 times less** with "rapid heal". Thus, "rapid heal" reduced the odds remaining unhealed to about 75% of what they would have been and reduced the odds by 25% of what they were in the control group.

When looking at RRs or ORs, always try and think:

- *Is it less than 1, more than 1, or equal to 1?*
- *What then does that tell us about events in the experimental group (are they happening less than, more than, or the same as in the control group)?*

This gives us a way of comparing what is happening in the "I" and "C" group of an RCT to see if the intervention of interest seems to have worked better, worse, or the same as the comparison group.

A word about confidence intervals

I also said in the hypothetical "rapid heal" example that after 6 weeks the RR was 0.8 with a **95% CI of 0.4 to 1.2.** So let's remind ourselves what a CI is and what it means.

As I said earlier in this chapter, if you think about an RCT and who is included, it is **not** the total population you are interested in; instead, it is a sample of that population and you hope that if you have selected a large random sample, it represents this population, and when you have randomly allocated to I and C and carried out a well-conducted unbiased trial, that what is found is an unbiased estimate of what is going on.

However, the RR value found for your sample is only a *point estimate* of what is going on. The 95% CI provides a range of numeric outcomes that we are reasonably confident includes the actual (population) result (Sheldon, 2008). So in our (hypothetical) example, the interval is saying that the RR would be as low as 0.4 or as high as 1.2. This range included the "no difference" estimate of 1 (remember that earlier I said if the **RR = 1,** it would tell us **events were happening at the SAME rate in both groups**), so this would NOT be a statistically significant answer. Therefore, with RRs or ORs, for a result to be statistically significant, you would **not** want to see the "no difference" result of 1 in the 95% CI.

Box 7.4   Interpretation of 95% CI

This explains how to interpret the first outcome of the risk of remaining unhealed after 6 weeks given as an **RR of 0.8 (see "blob" on the following diagram) with a 95% CI of 0.4 to 1.2 (see arrows on diagram).** Although initially it looked like "rapid heal" reduced the risk of remaining unhealed after 6 weeks, WHEN THE CONFIDENCE INTERVAL WAS TAKEN INTO ACCOUNT, because the range included the "no difference value" of 1, it was considered a not statistically significant finding. This is why it is important to always present CIs with the effect measure.

I have found students find it easier to visualize this by drawing a number line, as shown in the following figure.

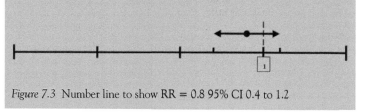

Figure 7.3 Number line to show RR = 0.8 95% CI 0.4 to 1.2

With these field examples, have a think if the outcomes of interest could be dichotomous.

Table 7.4 Questions from the different branches of nursing regarding "is there a cause and effect" relationship

Adult field example: Does **topical negative pressure** heal chronic wounds?	Child field example: Does **emollient cream** resolve childhood eczema?
Mental health field example: Do **coping strategies** reduce stress in carers of relatives with dementia?	Learning disabilities field example: Does **exercise** reduce anxiety in people with a learning disability?

Box 7.5 Hypothetical trial looking at the effect of honey on presence or absence of oral mucositis at 1 week

You saw how a PICO for this was constructed, how a basic search strategy could be constructed, how a pertinent RCT might look, and how you might critically appraise it looking for sources of bias, and now I am asking you to imagine you are reading the results and seeing if the authors have analysed the findings using appropriate effect measures and if you can interpret them.

Outcome 1: Looked at how many people have oral mucositis after 1 week

Table 7.5 2 × 2 table

	Event	No Event	Total
	Presence of oral mucositis after 1 week	Absence of oral mucositis after 1 week	
Experimental + honey	40	60	100
Control − saline	50	50	100

$$R_E = \frac{\text{having the event (presence of oral mucositis after 1 week)}}{\text{total}}$$

$$R_E = 40/100$$

$$R_C = \frac{\text{having the event (presence of oral mucositis after 1 week)}}{\text{total}}$$

$$R_C = 50/100$$

To compare the two risks or likelihoods, we can calculate a risk ratio (RR):

$$RR = \frac{40/100}{50/100}$$

$$RR = 0.8$$

So it is your turn to ask yourself: what does this mean?

Whenever you see an RR, ask yourselves is the RR <1, >1, or =1 and what does this tell us about events happening in the experimental group?

Box 7.6   Interpretation of RR

In this case the RR is less than 1 and that tells us Events (presence of oral mucositis after 1 week) are happening less in the experimental I/(honey) group than in the control (C/saline) group: little number (40/100) divided by a bigger number (50/100) gives us a number less than 1. Essentially, your **risk/likelihood** of the presence of oral mucositis after 1 week with this **hypothetical** data is essentially **0.8 times less** with honey. Honey reduced the risk to 80% of what it would have been, or honey reduced the risk by 20% of what it was in the control group.

Remember, though, this is just one point estimate from one sample. Let's imagine the hypothetical 95% CI was given as 0.7 to 0.9. So now it is your turn to interpret what this means.

Box 7.7   Interpretation of 95% CI

So in this example we see that the risk of oral mucositis after 1 week is given as an RR of 0.8 (**see "blob" on diagram that follows**) with a 95% CI, which could be as low as 0.7 or as high as 0.9 (**see arrows on diagram**). At the upper end of the range, it is still less than 1, implying less of the event (oral mucositis) with honey than with the saline. Because the 95% CI does NOT include the "no difference" RR result of 1 in the CI range, this **would** be considered a statistically significant answer – remember, though, this is a hypothetical example!

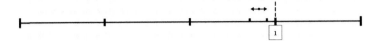

Figure 7.4 Number line to show RR = 0.8 and 95% CI 0.7 to 0.9

Table 7.6 Interpreting dichotomous measures of effectiveness

RR value	95% CI	Statistically significant? (tip: significant if the 95% CI did NOT include the "no difference" result value of 1)
0.99	0.80–1.18	no
2.0	1.8–2.2	yes
1.5	1.3–1.7	yes
0.03	0.01–0.05	yes
1.1	0.5–1.6	no

Summary

- As well as being able to judge if research designs are ethical and trustworthy, you need to understand if how the data has been collected and analysed is APPROPRIATE and if you can INTERPRET the results.
- When an RCT is carried out, essentially we are trying to determine what is happening in the experimental/I group in comparison to the control/C group to see if the intervention/I is having any effect on the outcome.
- We wish to infer things from the sample to the target population, and to do that we can use hypothesis testing using p values or estimation using CIs – we have focused on the latter method in this chapter (Freeman & Julious, 2021).
- If someone can be in one of two states (but not both at the same time), at the end of the study period these are known as **binary or dichotomous outcomes** e.g. unhealed/healed, infected/not infected.

- A way of comparing what is going on in the experimental group compared to the comparison group is to calculate a **risk** of poor outcome in each group.
- A **risk ratio** compares your risk in the experimental group **divided** by your risk in the comparison group. This is an <u>effect measure</u>.
- An RR greater than 1 indicates the event/outcome is happening more in the experimental group, an RR less than 1 indicates the event/outcome is happening less in the experimental group, and an RR = 1 indicates the event/outcome is happening the same in both groups.
- Another way of comparing what is going on in the experimental group compared to the comparison group is to calculate your **odds** of poor outcome in each group.
- An **odds ratio** compares your odds in the experimental group **divided** by your odds in the comparison group. This is also an <u>effect measure</u>.
- An odds ratio greater than 1 indicates greater odds of the event/outcome in the experimental group, an odds ratio less than 1 indicates smaller odds of the event/outcome in the experimental group, and an odds ratio = 1 indicates no difference in odds for the event/outcome between the two groups.
- When interpreting any effect measure initially, it might look like the intervention was effective, but you must consider:

    - The role of any **bias**.
    - This is one point estimate from one sample rather than a plausible range within which the true effect measure could lie with a certain degree of probability, so a **confidence interval** is needed to determine statistical significance or not.

- **For risk ratios or odds ratios, the "no difference" value is 1**, so if the 95% CI includes **1** it is considered NOT statistically significant; if the 95% CI does NOT include **1** it IS considered statistically significant. (Remember you could be wrong 5% of the time, though.)
- Appreciating this is further developing your critical appraisal and interpretive skills of quantitative data analysis for dichotomous outcomes.

References

Alderson P, Green S (Eds) (2002) Chapter 11. In *Cochrane Collaboration Open Learning Material for Reviewers*. https://www.cochrane-net.org/open-learning/PDF/Openlearning-full.pdf?msclkid=1eaf5a43cecc11ecbd74b56 48ff2e12c. Accessed on 20/01/2021.

Banerjee A, Chitnis UB, Jadhav SL, Bhawalkar JS, Chaudhury S. (2009) Hypothesis testing, type I and type II errors. *Industrial Psychiatry Journal*; *18*(2): 127–131. doi: 10.4103/0972-6748.62274

Breakwell GM, Hammond S, Fife-Schaw. (1995) *Research Methods in Psychology*. London, Thousand Oaks and New Delhi: Sage Publications.

Clegg F. (1990) *Simple Statistics. A Course Book for the Social Scientists*. Cambridge: Cambridge University Press.

Cumming G. (2014) The new statistics why and how. *Psychological Science*; *25*(1): 7–29.

Devore, Jay L. (2008) *Probability and Statistics for Engineering and the Sciences*. 7th edn. Belmont CA: Brooks/Cole Cengage Learning.

du Prel JB, Hommel G, Röhrig B, Blettner M. (2009) Confidence interval or p-value? Part 4 of a series on evaluation of scientific publications. *Deutsches Arzteblatt International*; *106*(19): 335–339. doi: 10.3238/arztebl.2009.0335

Freeman JV, Julious SA. *Hypothesis Testing and Estimation*. Medical Statistics Group, School of Health and Related Research, University of Sheffield, UK. www.sheffield.ac.uk/polopoly_fs/1.43993!/file/Scope-tutorial-4.pdf. Accessed on 26/10/2021.

Gardner MJ, Altman, DG. (1986) Confidence intervals rather than P values: estimation rather than hypothesis testing. *British Medical Journal (Clinical Research Ed.)*, -03; *292*(6522): 746–750.

Gates S. Blog. (2016) *The Probability That the Results Are Due to Chance*. 12/11/2016, Evidence-based everything (warwick.ac.uk)

Higgins JPT, Li T, Deeks JJ. (2021) Chapter 6: Choosing effect measures and computing estimates of effect. In Higgins JPT, Thomas J, Chandler J, Cumpston M, Li T, Page MJ, Welch VA (Eds) *Cochrane Handbook for Systematic Reviews of Interventions Version 6.2* (updated February 2021). www.training.cochrane.org/handbook.

McCormack J, Vandermeer B, Allan GM. (2013) How confidence intervals become confusion intervals. *BMC Medical Research Methodology*; *13*(1). https://link.gale.com/apps/doc/A534587395/AONE?u=uce&sid=bookmark-AONE&xid=25eb73fc. Accessed on 18/09/2021.

Sheldon TA. (2008) Chapter 12: Estimating treatment effects: Real or the result of chance? In Cullum N, Ciliska D, Haynes RB, Marks S (Eds)

Evidence Based Nursing: An Introduction (p. 86). Oxford: Blackwell Publishing Ltd.

Wilkinson M. (2013) Testing the null hypothesis: The forgotten legacy of Karl Popper? *Journal of Sports Science;* 31(9): 919–920. doi: 10.1080/02640414.2012.753636. Epub 2012 December 19. PMID: 23249368.

8 What are effect measures for continuous outcomes?

Consider again our trial looking at our fictitious product "rapid heal" on outcome 2. Remember we are still focusing on whether the data collected and analysed is appropriate and if you can interpret the results. In this chapter we are focusing on when data collected is <u>continuous</u> – see the section highlighted in   later.

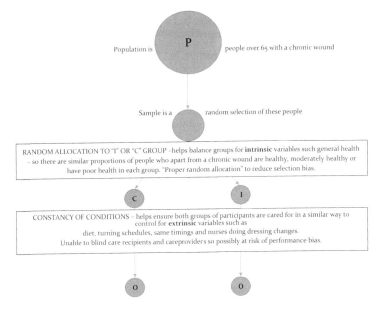

Figure 8.1 "Rapid heal" RCT representation

DOI: 10.4324/9781003156017-11

Data analyst is blinded to reduce detection bias. All patients are followed up to reduce attrition bias.

1.   **In relation to wounds remaining unhealed at 6 weeks,** the authors have presented a **risk ratio of 0.8 with a 95% confidence interval of 0.4 to 1.2.**
2.   **In relation to the average reduction in wound surface area at 2 weeks,** they have presented this as a **mean difference of 1.3 cm² with a 95% confidence interval of –0.1 cm² to 2.7 cm².**

Again don't worry if you don't understand these terms yet – the figures in the orange box are also <u>effect measures</u> – and we will go over the orange figures in this chapter.

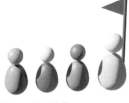

Figure 8.2 Follow me

Box 8.1   Continuous outcomes

Again, this may mean very little to you at present, but bear with me – I am again going to guide you through it so you can see:

a)   if the analysis is APPROPRIATE and
b)   if you can INTERPRET the results

So in this chapter we are focusing on whether our fictitious dressing "rapid heal" is having any effect on chronic wound healing vs. alternative dressing on average reduction in wound surface area at 2 weeks.

Mean differences

As I said earlier, when an RCT is carried out, essentially we are trying to determine what is happening in the experimental/I group in comparison to the control/C group to see if the intervention/I is having any effect on the outcome, and we hope to generalise these findings to a target population. For this we need **effect measures**, which as I said previously Higgins and Deeks define as statistical constructs that compare outcome data between two groups. Effect measures can broadly be divided into **ratio** measures (dealt with in the previous chapter) and **difference** measures (which we shall deal with in this chapter) (Higgins & Deeks, 2021).

So in our example, is "rapid heal" having any effect on chronic wound healing vs. an alternative dressing used for chronic wounds on the average reduction in wound surface area at 2 weeks? There are three common "averages" – the mean, median, and mode – and many people use the terms "average" and "mean" interchangeably, as I am doing here.

Mean difference

Box 8.2 Hypothetical trial looking at the effect of "rapid heal" on the average reduction in wound surface area at 2 weeks

So considering the second outcome of interest, you need to understand that this is a <u>continuous</u> outcome – "continuous data are data from outcomes measured on a continuous scale (for example blood pressure)" (Alderson & Green, 2002), height, weight, wound surface area.

We can look at the average/mean wound surface area reduction in the experimental/I/"rapid heal" group? Let's call this MeanE.

We can look at the average/mean wound surface area reduction in the control/C/alternative dressing group. Let's call this MeanC.

Here we have two means: MeanE and MeanC.

A way of comparing these two means is to **subtract** M_E by M_C – this is called a **mean difference** (by convention, the mean difference is calculated by subtracting the mean score for the control group from the mean score for the experimental group: M_E minus M_C) (Glen, 2021, Harris & Taylor, 2014) and this is also an <u>effect measure</u>.

So let's imagine:

In the experimental/I/"rapid heal" group, the mean reduction in wound surface area at 2 weeks was 3 cm^2.

In the control/C/alternative dressing group, the mean reduction in wound surface area at 2 weeks was 1.7cm^2.

Then the mean difference would be MeanE minus MeanC = 3 minus 1.7 = 1.3cm^2.

If the mean difference is >0, it tells us more of the thing is happening in the
experimental/I/"rapid heal" group, e.g. if MeanE – MeanC was 10 cm^2 minus 5 cm^2 = 5 cm^2).

If the mean difference was <0, it would tell us less of the thing is happening in the
experimental/I/"rapid heal group, e.g. if MeanE – MeanC was 5 cm^2 minus 10 cm^2 = –5 cm^2.

If the mean difference was = 0, it would tell us the thing was happening the SAME in both groups, e.g. if MeanE – MeanC was 10 cm^2 minus 10 cm^2 = 0. This would indicate **NO DIFFERENCE** between the two groups/interventions.

Box 8.3   Interpretation of the mean difference

In this case the **mean difference is 1.3 cm^2, which is >0 and tells us more of the thing is happening in the** experimental/I/"rapid heal" group (MeanE – MeanC was 3 cm^2 minus 1.7 cm^2 = 1.3 cm^2). Essentially, on average, it appears that wounds in the group receiving the fictitious "rapid heal" dressing had a reduction in wound surface area by 1.3cm^2 more than those receiving the control dressing.

Standardised mean differences should be used when studies assess the same outcomes but measure using different scales (Boland et al, 2014, p. 107).

A word about confidence intervals

I also said in the hypothetical "rapid heal" example that after 2 weeks the mean difference in wound surface area was 1.3 cm^2 with a **95%**

confidence interval of –0.1cm^2 to 2.7cm^2. So what is this and what does it mean?

If as I said earlier you think about an RCT and who is included, it is not the total population of people you are interested in – instead, it is a **sample** of that population, and you hope that if you have selected a large random sample, it represents this population, and when you have randomly allocated to "I" and "C" and carried out a well-conducted unbiased trial, that what is found is an unbiased estimate of what is going on.

But the mean difference value found for your sample is again a *point estimate* of what is going on. The 95% confidence interval provides a range of numeric outcomes (an *interval estimate*) that we are reasonably confident includes the actual (population) result (Sheldon, 2008). So in our hypothetical example, the interval is saying that the mean difference could be -0.1 cm^2 to 2.7 cm^2. This range included the "no difference" estimate of zero (remember that earlier I said if the **mean difference = 0, it would tell us the thing being measured –in this example, mean reduction in wound surface area – was happening by the SAME amount in both groups**). This would indicate **NO DIFFERENCE** between the two groups/interventions. Therefore, with mean differences, for a result to be statistically significant, you would **not** want to see the "no difference" result of zero in the 95% confidence interval.

Box 8.4   Interpretation of the 95% CI

This explains how to interpret the average reduction in wound surface area at 2 weeks given as a **mean difference of 1.3 cm^2 (see the "blob" on the diagram later) with a 95% confidence interval of –0.1cm^2 to 2.7cm^2 (see arrows on the diagram)**. Although initially it looked like the "rapid heal" increased the mean reduction in wound surface area at 2 weeks, WHEN THE CONFIDENCE INTERVAL WAS TAKEN INTO ACCOUNT, because the range included the "no difference" value of zero, it was considered a not statistically significant finding. This is why it is important to always present confidence intervals with the effect measure.

Again we can use a number line to visualize this, as shown in the figure.

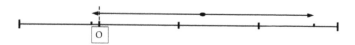

Figure 8.3 Number line to show MD = 1.3 95% CI –0.1 to 2.7

So let us see if you can apply this. Remember the **hypothetical** RCT examining the effect of honey on oral mucositis in patients? You saw how a PICO for this was constructed, how a basic search strategy could be constructed, how a pertinent RCT might look, and how you might critically appraise it looking for sources of bias, and now I am asking you to imagine you are reading the results and seeing if they have analysed the findings using appropriate effect measures and if you can interpret them.

Outcome 2: the average pain score after 1 week, which we shall deal with in this chapter.

Mean difference

> **Box 8.5   Hypothetical trial looking at the effect of honey on the average pain score after 1 week**
>
> So, focusing on the second outcome of interest – the average pain score at 1 week (with 0 representing no pain and 10 representing severe pain) – you need to understand that this is a <u>continuous</u> outcome. Some researchers treat it as if measuring on a 10-cm visual analogue (VA) scale.

We can look at the average/mean pain score in the experimental/ I/"rapid heal" group. Let's call this MeanE. We can look at the average/mean pain score in the control/C/alternative dressing group? Let's call this MeanC.

Here we have two means: MeanE and MeanC. A way of comparing these two means is to subtract M_E by M_C – this is called a **mean difference** (MD).

So let's imagine:

In the experimental/I/"honey" group, the mean pain score at 1 week was 4 on a 10-cm VA pain scale. In the control/C/saline group, the mean pain score at 1 week was 6 on a 10-cm VA pain scale. Then the MD would be MeanE minus MeanC = 4 minus 6 = –2 cm.

Whenever you see the MD, ask yourselves: is the MD greater than zero, less than zero, or is the MD equal to zero, and what does this tell us about what is happening in the experimental/honey group?

Box 8.6 Interpretation of the mean difference

In this case the **MD is –2 cm, which is <0 and tells us less of the thing is happening in** the experimental/I/"honey" group (MeanE – Mean C is 4 – 6 = –2). Essentially, on average, it appears that in this hypothetical trial patients in the group receiving honey experienced a lower mean pain score (by 2 cm) than those receiving the saline in relation to their oral mucositis.

Remember, though, this is just one point estimate from one sample. Let's imagine in the hypothetical honey example that after 1 week the MD in pain scores was –2 cm with a 95% confidence interval (CI) of –1.5 to –2.5 cm. So now it is your turn to interpret what this means.

Box 8.7 Interpretation of the 95% CI

This explains how to interpret the difference in mean pain scores at 1 week given as an **MD of –2 cm (see "blob" on diagram later) with a 95% CI of –1.5 to –2.5 cm (see arrows on diagram)**. Initially it looked like the honey reduced the pain score at 1 week and WHEN THE CONFIDENCE INTERVAL WAS TAKEN INTO ACCOUNT, because the range DID NOT include the "no difference" value of zero, it would be considered a statistically significant finding. This is why it is important to always present CIs with the effect measure. Remember, though, this is a hypothetical example!

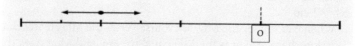

Figure 8.4 Number line to show MD = –2 95% CI –1.5 to –2.5

Table 8.1 Interpreting continuous measures of effectiveness

Mean difference value	95% confidence interval	Statistically significant? (tip: significant if the 95% CI did NOT include the "no difference" result value of 0)
–3	–1 to –5	Yes
1	–1 to 3	No
1.5	1.3 to 1.7	Yes
0.03	–0.01 to 0.07	No
7	4 to 10	Yes

Summary

- As stated in the previous chapter, as well as being able to judge if research designs are trustworthy, you need to understand if how the data has been collected and analysed is APPROPRIATE and if you can INTERPRET the results.
- When an RCT is carried out, essentially we are trying to determine what is happening in the experimental/I group in comparison to the control/C group to see if the intervention/I is having any effect on the outcome.
- We wish to infer things from the sample to the target population, and to do that we can use hypothesis testing and p values, or estimation based on effect sizes and confidence intervals. We have

focused on the latter method in this chapter (Freeman & Julious, 2021).

- A **continuous** variable refers to the numerical variable whose value is attained by measuring height, weight, and reduction in wound surface area, for example.
- A way of comparing what is going on in the experimental group compared to the comparison group is to calculate means for both groups and subtract the mean of the control group from the mean of the experimental group to find the **mean difference (MeanE minus MeanC)**. This is an effect measure.
- If the MD is >0, it tells us more of the thing is happening in the experimental/I group, if the mean difference is <0, it tells us less of the thing is happening in the experimental/I group, and if the mean difference is = 0, it tells us the thing is happening the SAME in both groups.
- When interpreting any effect measure, initially it might look like the intervention was effective, but you must consider:

    - The role of any **bias**.
    - This is one point estimate from one sample rather than a plausible range within which the true effect measure could lie with a certain degree of probability, so **a confidence interval is needed to determine statistical significance or not**.

- **For MDs (and standardised MDs), the "no difference" value is 0**, so if the 95% CI includes 0, it is considered NOT statistically significant; if the 95% CI does NOT include 0, it IS considered statistically significant. (Remember you could be wrong 5% of the time, though.)
- Appreciating this is further developing your critical appraisal and interpretive skills of quantitative data analysis for continuous outcomes.

References

Alderson P, Green S (Eds) (2002) Chapter 11. In *Cochrane Collaboration Open Learning Material for Reviewers*. https://www.cochrane-net.org/open-learning/PDF/Openlearning-full.pdf?msclkid=1eaf5a43cecc11ecbd74b56 48ff2e12c. Accessed on 20/01/2021.

Boland A, Cherry MG, Dickson R. (2014) *Doing a Systematic Review. A Student's Guide*. London: Sage Publications Ltd.

Freeman JV, Julious SA. *Hypothesis Testing and Estimation*. Medical Statistics Group, School of Health and Related Research, University of Sheffield, UK.   www.sheffield.ac.uk/polopoly_fs/1.43993!/file/Scope-tutorial-4.pdf. Accessed on 26/10/2021.

Glen S. (2021) *Mean Difference/Difference in Means (MD)*. From StatisticsHowTo.com: Elementary Statistics for the rest of us! www.statisticshowto.com/mean-difference/. Accessed on 08/11/2021.

Harris M, Taylor G. (2014) *Medical Statistics Made Easy*. Banbury: Scion Publishing Ltd.

Higgins JPT, Li T, Deeks JJ. (2021) Chapter 6: Choosing effect measures and computing estimates of effect. In Higgins JPT, Thomas J, Chandler J, Cumpston M, Li T, Page MJ, Welch VA (Eds) *Cochrane Handbook for Systematic Reviews of Interventions Version 6.2* (updated February 2021). www.training.cochrane.org/handbook.

Sheldon TA. (2008) Chapter 12: Estimating treatment effects: Real or the result of chance? In Cullum N, Ciliska D, Haynes RB, Marks S (Eds) *Evidence Based Nursing: An Introduction* (p. 86). Oxford: Blackwell Publishing Ltd.

9 How do you critically appraise quantitative evidence such as RCTs?

Table 9.1 Step 3

	3. Critically appraise the quantitative evidence

Ok – you deserve a pat on the back if you have managed to stick with me so far!

- At this point you have learned how to put a good research question together – be it quantitative or qualitative.
- You have learned how to put a good search strategy together to search for evidence – be it quantitative or qualitative.
- You have learned about the characteristics of quantitative randomised controlled trials (RCTs), which try to establish causation, and quantitative non-randomised studies (NRSs), namely quasi-experiments, cohort, and case-control quantitative research designs, which look for association.
- You have been introduced to the idea of how dichotomous quantitative data from such designs can be analysed and how this is interpreted (namely risk ratios, odds ratios, and confidence intervals).
- You have been introduced to the idea of how continuous quantitative data from such designs can be analysed and how this is interpreted (namely mean differences and confidence intervals).

DOI: 10.4324/9781003156017-12

- Now you are ready for the next **(third) step of the EBP process**, which is to **critically appraise** such quantitative designs.
- Remember "**critical appraisal** is the process of carefully and systematically examining research to judge its trustworthiness, and its value and relevance in a particular context" (Burls, 2009).

In this chapter I will introduce you to some guidance and tools used by researchers to essentially make a judgement of whether the quantitative evidence found is trustworthy. You will recognize features that we have already covered in previous chapters, and you will realise you are much more than halfway there and your hard work is paying off and you are engaging in the process of critically appraising quantitative research already!

Consider the work you have done so far regarding the hypothetical "honey trial" in terms of constructing a question, a search strategy, understanding the features of a hypothetical RCT where bias could have been minimised, and understanding how the hypothetical data was collected and analysed. I have summarised those things here before we consider tools for appraisal.

Table 9.2 Summary of work done so far regarding the hypothetical "honey trial"

ACP question:
In adults with radiation-induced oral mucositis, what is the effect of honey compared to 0.9% saline rinse on the presence of oral mucositis and pain score?

P	Adult patients with radiation-induced oral mucositis
I	Pure natural honey rinse
C	Routine mouth care by 0.9% saline rinse
O	The presence or absence of oral mucositis, pain score
D	This is a "what works" type question requiring RCTs to answer it

Sample search strategy:				
P #1 Adults with radiation therapy OR Radiotherapy OR Radiation-induced oral mucositis	I #2 Honey OR Topical honey OR Natural honey OR Pure natural honey OR Honey rinse	C Saline rinse	O Grade of oral mucositis OR Pain score	D #3 SR OR RCTs

(Continued)

Table 9.2 (Continued)

#1 **AND** #2 **AND** #3 would provide a basic search strategy for evidence on honey (and any other names for it) for adult patients with radiation-induced oral mucositis (and any other terms for it) from appropriate research designs that consider "what works best".

Remember previously I asked you to imagine you have found a relevant trial/ RCT using your search strategy and you are starting to look at **the characteristics and underpinning philosophy of this quantitative RCT research design.**

The hypothetical trial should have features built in to minimize bias where possible. "P" is the population of people with oral mucositis, "I" is the honey, "C" is the saline, and "O" is having/not having oral mucositis at week 1 and the pain scale score at week 1:

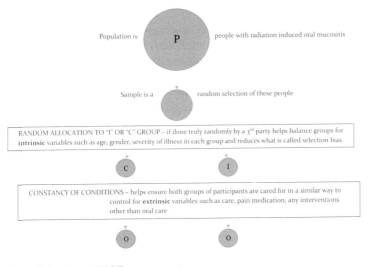

Figure 9.1 "Honey" RCT representation

Risk of bias assessment:

Random allocation to honey or saline by a third party would prevent any influence by the researcher of how people were allocated to groups, thus reducing **selection bias**. If possible, blinding care recipients and care providers to whether patients had received honey or saline would reduce **performance bias**, but in truth this would have been difficult since honey and saline look and feel different. So the study would possibly be at risk of performance bias – if people believe they are having a new treatment, they might report less pain, for example, one of the outcomes.

The person grading the oral mucositis would not have needed to know who had received honey or saline and so could assess it essentially blinded – this would reduce **detection bias**.

Blinding at all these three points is sometimes referred to as triple blinding.

Explaining/accounting for why any patients had dropped out with reasons would help reduce **attrition bias**.

1. For the presence of oral mucositis after 1 week, results are given as **a risk ratio of 0.8 with a 95% confidence interval of 0.7 to 0.9 – a statistically significant reduction.**
2. The difference in mean pain scores at 1 week is given as a **mean difference of –2 with honey and a 95% confidence interval of –1.5 to –2.5 – another statistically significant reduction.**

Is this study (albeit hypothetical) trustworthy? Before using any appraisal tools, I encourage my students to familiarise themselves with the **CONSORT** statement. This was written by a group of methodologists trying to encourage research authors to write up their RCTs better explaining in points 3 to 12 of their checklist WHAT methodological features are important and WHY (Moher et al, 2010). This was so readers (and systematic reviewers) would have sufficient methodological detail to appraise the trial and therefore make a judgement of its **internal validity** – its ability to show X was causing Y (if such a relationship was present) and thus how trustworthy the trial seemed.

Box 9.1 Features the Consort document (Moher et al, 2010) states it is important to describe

The trial **Design** so it could be quickly identified e.g. as an RCT in a search.

The **Participants** and settings to know who the findings could be generalised to.

The **Interventions** and **Counter-interventions** so sufficient detail is available for replication in further trials if necessary.

The **pre-specified** **Outcomes** and the instruments used to measure them to ensure they get reported on in the write-up and the tools' reliability and validity can be considered.

Do you recognize that this is PICOD?

How sample size was determined – There are calculations that can be done to determine the sample size required "to have a higher likelihood of showing a clinical difference of a certain size as statistically significant – if it really exists" (Moher et al, 2010).

Any interim analysis or stopping guidance – If the intervention was having a good or a bad effect, the study would need to be ended early for ethical reasons (Moher et al, 2010). So rather than analysing results at the end of the study, the data is analysed as it comes in so any significant good or bad outcomes can be detected sooner rather than later. This is better done by an independent third party.

VERY IMPORTANT is the reporting of the random assignment to I or C in terms of the sequence generation, the allocation concealment mechanism, and the implementation. CONSORT says that separate people should be involved with these three steps (Moher et al, 2010).

Remember we talked about reducing selection bias earlier?

Blinding refers to withholding information about the assigned interventions from people involved in the trial who may potentially be influenced by this knowledge (Moher et al, 2010) which means blinding of participants (care recipients) and care providers and data analysts where possible.

Remember we talked about reducing performance and detection bias before?

Statistical analysis – Statistical methods should be described with sufficient detail so that someone else would come up with the same results if they were to carry out the analysis. Along with an estimate of the treatment effect (effect measure) should be a confidence interval, which indicates a plausible range within which the true effect measure could lie with a certain degree of probability.

Remember we talked about effect measures for dichotomous and continuous outcomes and that confidence intervals should be reported?

Cochrane Risk of Bias tool

In brief, the Cochrane Risk of Bias (ROB) tool (Higgins et al, 2011) involves assessing studies for risk of bias arising from selection, performance, detection, attrition, reporting, or other sources. You will see in later chapters that this tool is used by Cochrane reviewers when critically appraising RCTs included in their SRs. There is an updated version of this tool – Cochrane ROB 2 (Sterne et al, 2019).

You will hopefully also recognise that we have already considered these sources of potential bias in the chapter on RCTs. When assessing studies for risk of bias, it needs to be done for each outcome/result, as bias can impact differently on different outcomes.

For example, let's imagine we have a study looking at an educational intervention to improve blood glucose levels in patients with type 2 diabetes. Let's say the outcomes of interest were blood glucose levels and compliance with a diabetic diet. If participants knew whether they were receiving the educational intervention or not, the study would be at risk of performance bias; however, the blood glucose levels in the short term wouldn't likely be affected by this lack of blinding, whereas the compliance with a diabetic diet could be affected. What if participants receiving the education had a desire to please the researcher, and it was this that led to a better compliance with a diabetic diet rather than the education itself?

I'm trying to explain in this example that the first outcome, i.e. blood glucose levels being physiological, would be less likely to be affected by performance bias, whereas the second outcome, i.e. compliance being more about someone's behaviour, could be more affected by performance bias.

Risk of bias in our hypothetical honey on oral mucositis trial using Cochrane's ROB tool

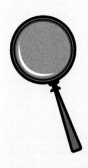

Users of the ROB tool not only have to look at the risk of bias but form a judgement as to whether for that particular source of bias there was a **low, high,** or **unclear** risk of bias backed up by a supportive statement for this judgement (Higgins et al, 2011).

So with our honey trial, for example, the Cochrane ROB tool asks for the author's judgement and a supportive comment for this judgment regarding selection, performance, detection, attrition, reporting, and any other sources of bias.

With selection bias, we could say it was a low risk of bias because participants had been randomly allocated to honey or saline using a computer-generated random sequence that was concealed and implemented by a third party.

However, for performance bias, we would have to say it was at high risk of bias because neither the care providers nor the care recipients were blind to the intervention – both would know whether patients were receiving honey or saline. There was probably a greater risk of performance bias in relation to the pain outcome, which relies on more subjective reporting than whether there was the presence or absence of mucositis, which could be determined more objectively.

With detection bias, we could say it was a low risk of this bias because the data analyst was blind to who had received honey or saline when assessing for the presence or absence of mucositis and pain.

With attrition bias, we could say it was at low risk of bias, as all participants were followed up.

The Critical Appraisal Skills Programme (CASP) tool for RCTs

This is a widely taught tool used to appraise RCTs that looks at study **quality** (the CASP tool for RCTs 2019). The core CASP checklists (RCT and systematic review) were based on *JAMA* "Users" guides to the medical literature 1994 (adapted from Guyatt GH, Sackett DL, and Cook DJ) (Guyatt et al, 2008). My students often use the Cochrane ROB tool or this tool when appraising RCTs in their background literature for their assignments.

Applying the CASP tool for RCTs to our hypothetical honey trial

The CASP tool for RCTs looks at quality and bias elements, so it asks things like whether the study asked a clearly focused question and whether it was an RCT. So being able to say what the PICO was helps determine if it asks a clearly focused question and identify if there was manipulation of an intervention, random allocation to groups, and control over intrinsic and extrinsic variables, which helps to determine if it was an RCT. The logic is that by ruling out other variables, one can be more confident about the relationship between the two variables of interest (the independent variable and the hypothesized dependent variable, or the I and the C – in this case the use of medical-grade honey vs. saline for 1 week on oral mucositis and pain).

Once it has been established that it is an RCT, more detailed questions follow regarding the design as to whether random allocation to groups was truly random to check for selection bias; whether the same care was provided to both groups (constancy of conditions); whether care providers, care recipients, and data analysts were blinded to assess for performance and detection bias; and whether all participants were accounted for at the end of the trial to assess for attrition bias.

Then questions regarding data collection and analysis follow as to whether all the participants had been followed up in the same way using valid and reliable tools and processes to measure outcomes, whether appropriate data analysis had been employed, and whether suitable effect measures and confidence intervals had been presented. So, for example, if one person assessed the patients with a reliable and valid instrument to measure pain – such as a visual analogue scale at the same time (after 1 week) in the same way – this would give confidence that data had been collected in the same way. If more than one person was collecting the data, their inter-rater reliability would have to have been checked. The CASP tool for RCTs also looks at whether a sample size calculation was carried out.

The CASP tool for RCTs asks how the results are presented and how precise they are. You will hopefully realise by now that this refers to effect measures such as mean differences and risk ratios/ odds ratios. Based on how precise an estimate is, confidence intervals should be reported.

The 95% confidence interval for the risk ratio (RR) of 0.8 was 0.7 to 0.9. This suggests that the risk of having oral mucositis at 1 week is statistically significantly smaller in the group given honey, as the interval does not incorporate the "no difference" result of 1.

The 95% confidence interval for the mean difference of –2 was –1.5 to –2.5 cm. Honey reduced the pain score at 1 week, and when the confidence interval was taken into account, because the interval did not include the "no difference" value of 0, it was considered a statistically significant finding too.

We would have to bear in mind that with this level of confidence, 5% of the time we could be wrong.

How can you use this in assignments?

Students are often asked to be critical rather than purely descriptive in their assignments, thus making a judgement about the trustworthiness of the research. You can see hopefully that if you applied the Cochrane ROB tool or the CASP tool for RCTs in the **hypothetical** honey trial, the findings indicate administering honey appears to significantly reduce the presence of oral mucositis and mean pain scores at 1 week among patients with radiation-induced oral mucositis. Remember whenever a trial is conducted, there are three possible explanations for the results: a) the findings are correct (truth), b) the findings represent random variation (chance), or c) they are influenced by systematic error (bias) (Moher et al, 2010, Mhaskar et al, 2009). We can check for inadequacies in the research design, data collection, and data analysis to look at b), for example, too small a sample size and c), steps taken to minimise the different sources of bias. So you might form a judgement if a sample size calculation had been performed whether it had an adequate sample size (to show a difference if there was one) and that the study was not at risk of selection bias, detection bias, or attrition bias but was at risk of performance bias. The analysis seemed appropriate, as effect measures including confidence intervals were presented. Because the outcomes were regarding presence or absence of mucositis, knowing whether you had received honey or saline would probably not have had an impact on this – but performance bias might be more of an issue when self-reporting on pain. What if the patient knew that honey was a new thing and wanted to please the researcher? So would you trust this study? Although the findings were statistically significant, were they clinically significant? Risk ratios are relative values – Were any absolute values provided? Would you change practice as a result? Including paragraphs like this in your work would get you points for demonstrating critical thinking.

How do you critically appraise quantitative evidence such as NRSs?

The STROBE statement (Vandenbroucke et al, 2007) was written by a group of methodologists a few years after CONSORT trying to encourage research authors to write up their NRSs better so readers (and reviewers) would have sufficient methodological detail to assess the risk of bias within NRS and therefore make a judgement of how trustworthy these studies seemed. Tools used to appraise NRSs include the Risk of Bias in NRS (ROBiNRS) tool (Sterne et al, 2016), the CASP tool for cohort studies, and the CASP tool for case-control studies (CASP for Cohort Studies, 2018, CASP for Case Control Studies, 2018).

<u>You could have a go at appraising the hypothetical SIDS case-control study using the ROBiNRS tool.</u>

Summary

- Critical appraisal is the process of carefully and systematically examining research to judge its trustworthiness and its value and relevance in a particular context (Burls, 2009).
- The CONSORT statement points 3 through 12 are useful to inform you WHAT needs to be included in a trial and WHY.
- You have already learned that an RCT is a research approach designed to answer a **"what works best"** question. It is the ONLY research design that features RANDOM ALLOCATION to groups, which helps to control for intrinsic variables and therefore for **selection bias**.
- The RCT should have constancy of conditions where possible for both groups to control for extrinsic variables.
- From a design point of view, blinding of care providers and care recipients to reduce performance bias, blinding of data analysts to reduce detection bias, and accounting for any withdrawals (and reasons) to reduce attrition bias would be desirable. This is not always possible, of course. The RCT authors should provide effect measures that include confidence intervals.
- In this chapter we have considered commonly used tools for appraisal of quantitative studies and applied two to our hypothetical honey trial.
- The Cochrane ROB tool is useful to look for potential sources of bias within a trial.
- The CASP tool for RCTs is useful to look for quality elements and some bias elements within a trial.
- The ROBiNRS tool is useful to look for potential sources of bias in NRSs.
- The CASP tools for cohort and case-control studies are useful to look for quality elements and bias elements, especially in relation to selection bias, as these studies lack random allocation.

- You would normally pick one tool to appraise an article and justify your choice.
- Remember in the previous chapters I mentioned it is very important to assess for bias before interpreting the results of a study. Would you trust the results if they came from a study full of bias?

References

Burls A. (2009) *What is Critical Appraisal?* The Bandolier Report. http://www. bandolier.org.uk/painres/download/whatis/What_is_critical_appraisal.pdf? msclkid=2ee70a20bdfe11ecaff1d5d9317b676b

Critical Appraisal Skills Programme. (2018a). *CASP Cohort Study Checklist.* https://casp-uk.b-cdn.net/wp-content/uploads/2018/01/CASP-Cohort-Study-Checklist_2018.pdf. Accessed on 12/10/2021.

Critical Appraisal Skills Programme. (2018b). *CASP Case Control Study Checklist.* https://casp-uk.b-cdn.net/wp-content/uploads/2018/03/CASP-Case-Control-Study-Checklist-2018_fillable_form.pdf. Accessed on 12/10/2021.

Critical Appraisal Skills Programme. (2019) *CASP Randomised Controlled Trials Checklist.* https://casp-uk.b-cdn.net/wp-content/uploads/2020/10/CASP_RCT_Checklist_PDF_Fillable_Form.pdf. Accessed on 12/10/2021.

Guyatt G, Rennie D, Meade M, Cook DJ. (2008) *Users Guides to the Medical Literature: Essentials of Evidence Based Clinical Practice.* 2nd edn. New York: McGraw Hill.

Higgins JPT, Altman DG, Gotzsche PC, Juni P, Moher D, Oxman AD. et al. (2011) The Cochrane collaboration's tool for assessing risk of bias in randomised trials. *BMJ*; 343: d5928. doi: 10.1136/bmj.d5928

Mhaskar R, Emmanuel P, Mishra S, Patel S, Naik E, Kumar A. (2009) Critical appraisal skills are essential to informed decision-making. *Indian Journal of Sexually Transmitted Diseases and AIDS*; 30(2): 112–119. doi: 10.4103/0253-7184.62770

Moher D, Hopewell S, Schulz KF, Montori V, Gøtzsche PC, Devereaux PJ, Elbourne D, Egger M, Altman DG. (2010) CONSORT 2010 explanation and elaboration: Updated guidelines for reporting parallel group randomised trials. *BMJ*; 340: c869.

Sterne JAC, Hernán MA, Reeves BC, Savović J, Berkman ND, Viswanathan M, Henry D, Altman DG, Ansari MT, Boutron I, Carpenter JR, Chan AW, Churchill R, Deeks JJ, Hróbjartsson A, Kirkham J, Jüni P, Loke YK, Pigott TD, Ramsay CR, Regidor D, Rothstein HR, Sandhu L, Santaguida PL, Schünemann HJ, Shea B, Shrier I, Tugwell P, Turner L, Valentine JC, Waddington H, Waters E, Wells GA, Whiting PF, Higgins JPT. (2016)

ROBINS-I: A tool for assessing risk of bias in non-randomized studies of interventions. *BMJ; 355*: i4919. doi: 10.1136/bmj.i4919.

Sterne JAC, Savovic J, Page MJ, Elbers RG, Blencowe NS, Boutron I, Cates CJ, Cheng H-Y, Corbett MS, Eldridge SM, Emberson JR, Hernán MA, Hopewell S, Hróbjartsson A, Junqueira DR, Jüni P, Kirkham J, Lasserson T, Li T, . . . Higgins JPT. (2019) RoB 2: A revised tool for assessing risk of bias in randomised trials. *BMJ; 366*(l4898). doi: 10.1136/bmj.l4898

Vandenbroucke JP, von Elm E, Altman DG, Gøtzsche PC, Mulrow CD, Pocock SJ, Poole C, Schlesselman JJ, Egger M. (2007) STROBE initiative. Strengthening the reporting of observational studies in epidemiology (STROBE): Explanation and elaboration. *PLoS Medicine, 16*;4(10): e297. doi: 10.1371/journal.pmed.0040297. PMID: 17941715; PMCID: PMC2020496.Strobe

10 Let's talk about characteristics of some qualitative designs – phenomenology, ethnography, and grounded theory

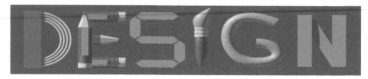

Figure 10.1 "Design" logo

As I said in Chapters 4 and 5, if you understand the characteristics of a design, you will better understand different research studies' methodological strengths and weaknesses. If you can recognise these strengths and weaknesses, you can start to critically appraise the studies. This important skill helps you judge whether a study's findings are trustworthy or not. As I said before, this can aid decision making. You can ask yourself whether you trust the results and would it impact on your practice.

Just as you did with quantitative studies, before you can learn about the process of appraising **qualitative** research studies, you need to learn about different qualitative research designs.

In previous chapters I have already mentioned if we want to know "how does it feel" researchers use a qualitative approach. And remember we can still use the research process as a guide.

1. Denzin and Lincoln describe qualitative research as "a set of interpretive, material practices that make the world visible. These practices transform the world. They turn the world into a series of representations, including field notes, interviews,

DOI: 10.4324/9781003156017-13

conversations, photographs, recordings and memos to self . . . qualitative researchers study things in their natural settings, attempting to make sense of or interpret phenomena in terms of the meanings people bring to them" (Denzin & Lincoln, 2005, p. 3).

2. It is an overarching term that includes a variety of approaches such as phenomenology, ethnography, and grounded theory that share some similarities but emphasise different aims and perspectives (Bhandari, 2020).

Table 10.1 Some qualitative research approaches

Phenomenology (has roots in psychology and philosophy)	This approach aims to describe and interpret people's lived experience.
	It seeks to uncover personal meaning, as "different people may consciously experience the world in quite diverse ways" (Polgar & Thomas, 1991, p. 98).
	<u>**Descriptive phenomenology**</u> was first developed by Husserl (Polit & Beck, 2018) in order to understand and define the phenomenon/experience and put forward the notion that one should "bracket", or "put aside the usual preconceptions and prejudices that influence every day perception . . . to uncover the pure constituents of conscious experience" (Polgar & Thomas, 1991, p. 98).
	<u>Interpretive phenomenology/hermeneutics</u> – Heidegger believed it was impossible to bracket one's "being in the world" (Polit & Beck, 2018, p. 188), and the researcher and the prior understanding of the researcher were also part of the interpretation that emerges from the analysis.
Ethnography (has roots in anthropology)	This approach aims to describe and interpret cultures in order to understand the way ideas, values, customs, beliefs, knowledge, behaviours, and activities of groups of people "guides their view of the world and the way they structure their experience" (Polit & Beck, 2018, p. 186).
	Researchers want to learn about the meanings a cultural group attaches to their knowledge, behaviours, and activities (Ploeg, 2008).
	They want to understand groups of people's worldview so they immerse themselves in groups or organisations to understand their cultures.

(Continued)

Table 10.1 (Continued)

Grounded theory (has roots in sociology)	This approach aims to collect rich data on a topic and develop theories inductively to discover social-psychological processes (Ploeg, 2008).
	Researchers try to account for people's actions from the perspective of those involved.
	It involves "the constant comparative method of coding and analysing data to develop concepts and the theoretical sampling method with cases selected purposively to refine the 'theory' previously developed" (Polgar & Thomas, 1991, p. 126).
Descriptive qualitative studies	No particular disciplinary or methodological roots, but employs the same data collection and data analysis methods.

▼

3. Each of these uses one or more of the data collection methods discussed in the table.

Table 10.2 Some qualitative data collection methods

In-depth interviews	Researchers record what is said in unstructured or semi-structured 1–1 conversation
Focus groups	Researchers record what is discussed in a facilitated discussion group
Observation	Researchers record what is seen/heard in detailed field notes – could be direct/indirect, unstructured or structured, overt/covert, and researcher is involved (emic) or more remote (etic)
Existing data	Researchers collect relevant textual, audio, or video material
Open-ended questionnaires	Researchers collect responses to open-ended questions

▼

4. There are several approaches to analysing qualitative data – they share similar processes but emphasise different concepts (Bhandari, 2020). Qualitative research produces a mass of descriptive data that the researcher must then try to interpret using systematic methods of transcribing, coding, and analysis of narrative (rather than numbers) to look for meaning (rather than relationships between variables).

Table 10.3 Some qualitative data analysis methods

Content analysis
Thematic analysis
Textual analysis
Discourse analysis

The researcher's analysis of the data is an interpretation or construction of the meaning of the participants' words or actions (Skodol Wilson, 1993). Sandelowski and Barroso (2003) state that "qualitative research findings are on a continuum indicating degrees of transformation of data during data analysis from description to interpretation". Descriptive phenomenology, content analysis, and thematic analysis might be considered by some as "low-level interpretation" compared to, say, interpretive phenomenology.

5. The final phase of the research process would be to report on what has been discovered about these people's reality of a particular situation.

Remember in earlier chapters we considered "how does it feel" so we are going to focus more now on phenomenology.

Box 10.1 Phenomenology definition

Phenomenology is described as "the study of human meanings and practices, with an emphasis on interpreting lived experience from narrative text" (Skodol Wilson, 1993, p. 236).

We are still going to critically examine this claim. But first let me teach you about the basic setup of such a study with this hypothetical scenario:

Qualitative scenario 1 – A research group has been asked to explore the research question "When family carers take care of a child with profound multiple learning disabilities, what are their experiences?" Because they wish to describe and interpret the lived experience of carers, they have adopted a phenomenological approach and have proceeded to set up the study.

Table 10.4 Basic steps in descriptive phenomenology	APPLIED TO HYPOTHETICAL "SCENARIO$_1$"
State the research purpose Remember I said earlier that with qualitative studies like grounded theory, it can be more theory-generating rather than hypothesis testing. With phenomenology, it is not about generating theory, but rather "transforming a lived experience into a textual expression that reflects something meaningful" (Skodol Wilson, 1993, p. 236).	Find out about the experiences of family carers when they take care of a child with profound multiple learning disabilities.
Decide the study design/ theoretical framework. In qualitative research there is no talk of independent and dependent variables. There is no attempt to exert control over the situation or on individuals, to randomise, or to use blinding, as you are not trying to establish cause and effect or association. The aim in qualitative research is different. A qualitative approach is characterised by the study of phenomena in its natural context. With phenomenology the aim is to uncover personal meaning, as "different people may consciously experience the world in quite diverse ways" (Polgar & Thomas, 1991, p. 98).	Use a phenomenological approach and follow the steps associated with such an approach. This is known as "methodological coherence" (Richards & Morse, 2007); e.g. with descriptive phenomenology, the researcher might use a reflexive diary (Polit & Beck) to try to bracket preconceptions or prejudices before and during the research processes.

(Continued)

Table 10.4 (Continued)

Identify the participants of interest and select a sample. In contrast to quantitative research, the aim is not to generalise findings from a representative random sample to a target population; rather, the aim here would to be to gather accounts from a purposive sample of individuals until no new information was obtained, which is known as data saturation. It is still useful to know how many participants were included to assess the breadth of perspectives included. **Describe the setting and the context** as it may show why people responded in a particular way.	After obtaining ethical approval to carry out the study, approach carers to explore their experiences of taking care of a child with multiple learning disabilities. Explain the purpose of the study, its benefits, risks, and the voluntary nature of taking part before obtaining their written informed consent. Participants needed to have experienced the phenomenon and be willing to talk about it in order to provide rich data. Provide characteristics of participants. Use pseudonyms to ensure anonymity of participants. When asking carers to open up about a potentially upsetting experience, ensure support mechanisms are in place.
Collect data through semi-structured or unstructured in-depth interviews. In contrast to quantitative research, rather than the data needing to be valid and reliable, the research language for appraising qualitative research is different – the data needs to be confirmable, credible, and dependable. It is for the reader to judge transferability to similar situations (Polit & Beck, 2018).	Conduct in-depth semi-structured interviews lasting e.g. 60–90 minutes in a quiet private space. Ask broad open questions to begin with such as "Please can you tell me about your experiences of taking care of your child?" Be guided by the carers' answers to ask more probing questions. Make explicit what questions and prompts were used. Audio-record the interviews. Consider if more interviews with the same or different carers need to be carried out.

(Continued)

Table 10.4 (Continued)

Analyse narrative using a qualitative framework such as thematic analysis. Colaizzi's method is widely used by nurse researchers (Colaizzi, 1978, Wirihana et al, 2018) and involves: "1. Reading and rereading the transcript 2. Extracting significant statements that pertain to the phenomenon 3. Formulating meanings from significant statements 4. Aggregating formulated meanings into theme clusters and themes 5. Developing an exhaustive description of the phenomenon's essential structure or essence 6. A description of fundamental structure of the phenomenon is subsequently generated 7. Validation of the findings of the study through participant feedback completes the analysis"	Carefully listen to and transcribe verbatim each interview after each session. Also refer to any field notes or notes of non-verbal expression to aid interpretations. Return the transcripts to participants to check it reflects what they said. Then read multiple times. Highlight "stand out" phrases that seem to be key to indicate the experience of caring in these circumstances. Formulate meanings from these and put together into theme clusters and themes. Thematic data saturation is reached when no new themes emerge from the collected data (Guest et al, 2020). Develop an exhaustive description of the essence of the experience. Obtain feedback from participants regarding researchers' interpretations so they can say if their own perceptions are represented.
Report on what has been discovered about these people's reality of this situation. Include selection of vivid extract examples.	Let's imagine analysis of the data identified three major thematic areas which described carers' experiences when looking after children with profound multiple learning disabilities: challenges caring for one's child and oneself, experiencing both hope and helplessness, and accessing information and support to deal with the complexities of caring. You would present these with relevant quotes. After exploring the experiences of carers of children with profound multiple learning disabilities, compare the results of the research study with other research literature.

If you remember before when discussing quantitative approaches such as RCTs, post-positivists recognise that human beings may introduce bias, so we have to take steps to minimise it to make a study more trustworthy. Likewise, because the qualitative researcher is sometimes referred to as the "instrument", "all observations, interpretations, [and] analyses are filtered through their own personal lens" (Bhandari, 2020). Thus qualitative researchers need to recognise how their values/beliefs might impact on the research process – a process known as reflexivity (Polit and Beck, 2018). In both quantitative and qualitative approaches we want to see what has been done to make the research more trustworthy.

Table 10.5 Quantitative and qualitative quality criteria

Here is a reminder of **QUANTITATIVE** Quality criteria: (Polit & Beck, 2018)		Now let us consider **QUALITATIVE** Quality criteria: Lincoln and Guba (1985), Guba and Lincoln (1994)
Objectivity – extent to which personal biases are removed and value-free info is gathered	*Remember e.g. with RCT use random allocation to groups to reduce selection bias, blinding of care recipients and care providers to reduce performance bias, blinding of data analysts to reduce detection bias, and accounting for all withdrawals to reduce attrition bias*	**Confirmability** – extent to which findings are based on study's participants and settings instead of researchers' biases
Internal validity – extent to which observed effects can be attributed to the presumed cause	*Remember e.g. with RCT – due to random allocation to control for intrinsic variables, constancy of conditions for both groups to control for extrinsic variables, and steps taken to minimise potential sources of bias – this design has high internal validity*	**Credibility** – extent to which study's findings are believable to others

(Continued)

Table 10.5 (Continued)

Reliability – extent to which findings are consistent if study was replicated	For example, with RCT is sufficient detail provided about the PICO elements, measuring instruments, and data analysis approach so study could be replicated?	Dependability – extent to which findings are consistent in relation to the context in which they were generated
External validity – extent to which findings can be generalised from sample to target population	For example, with RCT, how representative is sample of target population – was it selected randomly?	Transferability – extent to which findings can be transferred/applied in other settings
		Authenticity – the extent to which researchers faithfully show a range of different realities and convey the feeling and tone of lives as they are lived

So here I am introducing you to Lincoln and Guba's idea that qualitative research can also be looked at critically, but using **different** criteria than is used for quantitative research (Lincoln & Guba, 1985, Guba & Lincoln, 1994). We will look at this in more detail in the next chapter.

Now instead of "when family carers take care of a child with profound multiple learning disabilities, what are their experiences?" – the "how does it feel" question just posed – consider the qualitative questions from the different nursing fields shown later.

Use Table 10.4 used for "scenario 1" to help you set up hypothetical qualitative studies for the field-specific examples provided. Think about any ethical issues that might arise from these in-depth conversations – such as talking about upsetting things and talking to children. Think about your own role, views, preconceptions, motivations, and how you would suspend these or acknowledge these (Tip:

reflexive journal). Think about how the experience could be captured by the interviewer in a confirmable, credible, dependable, and potentially transferable way (Tip: field notes describing the context, taking note of non-verbal communication, going back to participants regarding the transcripts or the generated themes).

Table 10.6 Examples of "how someone feels" questions from the four nursing fields

Adult field example: What is the impact of a non-healing venous leg ulcer in adults?	Child field example: What is the impact of repeated surgeries in children?
Mental health field example: What is the impact of repeated miscarriages in women?	Learning disabilities field example: What is the impact on family carers of caring for a child with profound multiple learning disabilities?

Table 10.7 Children's nurse **"how does it feel"** question

Children's nurse question:
What are parents' perceptions of non-pharmacological interventions for managing their children's pain post-elective surgery?
Use Table 10.4 for "scenario 1" to help you set up a hypothetical qualitative study for the "how does it feel" research question. Have a go before looking.

Table 10.8 Basic steps in descriptive phenomenology applied to HYPOTHETICAL "scenario 2"

State the research purpose.	Explore parents' perceptions of non-pharmacological interventions for managing their children's pain post-elective surgery.
Decide the study design/theoretical framework.	Use a phenomenological study and follow the steps associated with such an approach – "methodological coherence" (Richards & Morse, 2007).

(*Continued*)

Table 10.8 (Continued)

Identify the participants of interest and select a sample. Describe the setting and the context.	After obtaining ethical approval to carry out the study, approach parents to explore their perceptions of non-pharmacological interventions for managing their children's pain post-elective surgery. Explain the purpose of the study, its benefits, risks, and the voluntary nature of taking part before obtaining their written informed consent. They needed to have experienced the phenomenon and be willing to talk about it in order to provide rich data. Provide characteristics of participants. Use pseudonyms to ensure the anonymity of participants. When asking parents to open up about a potentially upsetting experience, ensure support mechanisms are in place.
Collect data through semi-structured or unstructured in-depth interviews.	Conduct in-depth semi-structured interviews lasting 30–60 minutes in a quiet private space. Ask broad open questions to begin with such as "Please can you describe your experience of managing your child's pain after surgery?" Be guided by the parents' answers to ask more probing questions. Make explicit what questions and prompts were used. Audio-record the interviews. Consider if more interviews with the same or different parents need to be carried out to reach data saturation.
Analyse narrative using a qualitative framework (Colaizzi, 1978, Wirihana et al, 2018).	Carefully listen to and transcribe verbatim each interview after each session. Also refer to any field notes or notes of non-verbal expression to aid interpretations. Return the transcripts to parents to check it reflects what they said. Then read multiple times. Highlight "stand out" phrases that seem to be key to indicate the experience of caring in these circumstances. Formulate meanings from these and put together into theme clusters and themes. Stop when no new themes emerge from the collected data. Develop an exhaustive description of the essence of the experience. Obtain feedback from parents regarding researchers' interpretations so they can say if their own perceptions are represented.

(Continued)

Table 10.8 (Continued)

Report on what has been discovered about these people's reality of this situation.	Let's imagine analysis of the data identified three major thematic areas which described parents' perceptions of non-pharmacological interventions for managing their children's pain post-elective surgery as feeling supported by professionals, familiarity with non-pharmacological interventions, and barriers to the use of non-pharmacological interventions. Present these with relevant quotes. After exploring the parents' perceptions compare the results of the research study with other research literature.

Table 10.9 Qualitative quality criteria

QUALITATIVE Quality criteria (Lincoln & Guba 1985), Guba and Lincoln (1994) for scenario 2	
Confirmability – extent to which findings are based on study's participants and settings instead of researchers' biases **Credibility** – extent to which study's findings are believable to others **Dependability** – extent to which findings are consistent in relation to the context in which they were generated **Transferability** – extent to which findings can be transferred/applied in other settings **Authenticity** – the extent to which researchers faithfully show a range of different realities and convey the feeling and tone of lives as they are lived	*Have a think about these for "scenario 2" – we will consider appraisal of such qualitative studies in more detail in the next chapter.*

Summary

- Qualitative research involves "interpretive practices" that claim to make the "world visible" (Denzin & Lincoln, 2005, p. 3).

- "It does not lend itself to empirical inference to a population as a whole, rather it allows researchers to generalise to a theoretical understanding of the phenomena being examined" (Ploeg, 2008, p. 54).
- Qualitative research is an overarching term that includes a variety of approaches such as phenomenology, ethnography, and grounded theory that share some similarities but emphasise different aims and perspectives.
- Similarities include naturalistic settings, small samples, non-numerical data, and the need for reflexivity.
- Phenomenology is a research approach designed to answer a **"how does it feel"** question – more specifically, "the study of human meanings and practices, with an emphasis on interpreting lived experience from narrative text" (Skodol Wilson, 1993, p. 236).
- You can ask yourself: is it confirmable – are findings based on the study's participants and settings instead of researchers' biases?
- Is it credible – is it believable to others?
- Is it dependable – are findings consistent in relation to the context in which they were generated?
- Is it transferable – can findings be transferred/applied in other settings?
- Is it authentic – does it convey how it is for those individuals?
- Ethical approval and informed consent is still vital for qualitative studies e.g. to ensure support mechanisms are in place if participants are asked about upsetting situations and that they know they have the right to remain anonymous, refuse to participate, and withdraw at any time without it affecting care.
- Appreciating this is further developing your critical appraisal skills.

References

Bhandari P. (2020) *An Introduction to Qualitative Research.* www.scribbr.com/methodology/qualitative-research/. Accessed on 10/11/2021.

Colaizzi P. (1978) Psychological research as the phenomenologist views it. In Vale RS, King M (Eds) *Existential-Phenomenological Alternatives for Psychology.* New York NY: Oxford University Press.

Denzin N, Lincoln Y. (Eds) (2005) *Handbook of Qualitative Research*. 3rd edn. Thousand Oaks, CA: Sage.

Guba E, Lincoln Y. (1994) Competing paradigms in qualitative research. In Denzin N, Lincoln Y (Eds) *Handbook of Qualitative Research* (pp. 105–117). Thousand Oaks, CA: Sage.

Guest G, Namey E, Chen M. (2020) A simple method to assess and report thematic saturation in qualitative research. *PLoS ONE*; *15*(5): e0232076. doi: 10.1371/journal.pone.0232076

Lincoln YS, Guba EG. (1985) *Naturalistic Inquiry*. Beverly Hills, CA: Sage.

Ploeg J. (2008) Identifying the best research design to fit the question. Part 2: Qualitative research. In Cullum N, Ciliska D, Haynes RB, Marks S (Eds) *Evidence Based Nursing: An Introduction* (p. 54). Oxford: Blackwell Publishing Ltd.

Polgar S, Thomas SA. (1991) *Introduction to Research in the Health Sciences*. 2nd edn. Melbourne; Edinburgh; London; New York: Churchill, Livingstone.

Polit DF, Beck CT. (2018) *Essentials of Nursing Research: Appraising Evidence for Nursing Practice*. 9th edn. Philadelphia. Wolters Kluwer.

Richards L, Morse JM. (2007) *Readme First for a User's Guide to Qualitative Methods*. Thousand Oaks: Sage Publications.

Sandelowski M, Barroso J. (2003) Classifying the findings in qualitative studies. *Qualitative Health Research*; *13*: 905–923.

Skodol Wilson H. (1993) *Introducing Research in Nursing*. 2nd edn. Canada: Addison Wesley Nursing – division of Benjamin/Cummings Publishing Company, Inc.

Wirihana L, Welch A, Williamson M, Christensen M, Bakon S, Craft J. (2018) Using Colaizzi's method of data analysis to explore the experiences of nurse academics teaching on satellite campuses. *Nurse Research*; *16*; *25*(4): 30–34. doi: 10.7748/nr.2018.e1516. PMID: 29546965.

11 How do you critically appraise qualitative evidence?

Table 11.1 Step 3

	3. Critically appraise the **qualitative** evidence

So to sum up at this point you have seen how to pose a question using PIO/PEO, construct a search strategy, and started to look at the characteristics of qualitative designs that your search might find. This is necessary before you can embark on the third step of the EBP process, which is to **critically appraise** such studies.

Remember "**critical appraisal** is the process of carefully and systematically examining research to judge its trustworthiness, and its value and relevance in a particular context" (Burls, 2009).

In this chapter I will further elaborate on Lincoln and Guba's quality criteria for qualitative research (1985) referred to in the previous chapter and introduce you to some popular strategies described by Polit and Beck (2018) to "strengthen integrity", followed by checklists and tools used by researchers to essentially make a judgement of whether the qualitative evidence found it trustworthy. Polit and Beck state that you "need to be persuaded about the researcher's conceptualization and to expect the researcher to present evidence with which to persuade you" (Polit & Beck, 2018, p. 304), but as Walsh points out, be aware there isn't a consensus amongst all qualitative researchers regarding qualitative critical appraisal (Walsh, 2006).

DOI: 10.4324/9781003156017-14

Table 11.2 Steps qualitative researchers can take for the different qualitative quality criteria

QUALITATIVE Quality criteria (Lincoln & Guba, 1985), Guba and Lincoln (1994):	*Steps qualitative researchers can take for the different quality criteria informed by Polit and Beck's quality enhancement strategies (Polit & Beck, 2018, pp. 296–304):*
Confirmability – extent to which findings are based on study's participants and settings instead of researchers' biases	➢ *Keep diary to reflect on process, researcher's role and influences, interviewer effect, and pre-understanding (**reflexivity**)* ➢ *Describe the personal characteristics of the researcher to give readers the ability to assess how these factors might have influenced the researchers' observations and interpretations* ➢ *Make explicit the relationship of the researcher with participants, as it can have an effect on the participants' responses and on the researchers' understanding of the phenomena* ➢ *Document steps and decisions taken and motives (**audit trail**)* ➢ *Discuss research process/findings with peers (**peer debriefing**) to ensure interpretations came from findings – not from your biases* ➢ *Include participant quotes to support researchers' interpretations to show results are grounded in the data rather than just viewpoints of the researchers*
Credibility – extent to which study's findings are believable to others	➢ *Use **multiple data sources*** ➢ *Method triangulation – might interview and observe* ➢ *Data triangulation – might have transcripts and field notes* ➢ *Investigator triangulation – might have two researchers coding the data* ➢ *Theory triangulation – might compare to someone else's theory on this topic* ➢ ***Prolonged engagement or persistent observation*** ➢ ***Respondent validation** of interview transcripts and themes* ➢ *Look for disconfirming cases*

(Continued)

Table 11.2 (Continued)

Dependability – extent to which findings are consistent in relation to the context in which they were generated	➤ **Member checks** – *to check researcher is reporting precisely what people say* ➤ *Collect data until no new data emerges* (**saturation**) ➤ *Iterative data collection (continually analyse to inform further data collection)* ➤ *Iterative data analysis (continually re-examine data using insights that emerge)* ➤ *Detailed audit trail documenting changes* ➤ *Provide direct quotes* ➤ *Ask yourself: would different interviewer asking same questions get same result?*
Transferability – extent to which findings can be transferred/applied in other settings	➤ *Give* **"thick"** *descriptions* – *include context and population characteristics to make findings meaningful to others* ➤ *Explain sampling strategy* ➤ *Check resonance (or not) with other literature in different settings* ➤ *Provide full theoretical framework for study* ➤ *It rests with the audience to judge transferability to similar situations based on the broad description of the findings (Polit & Beck, 2018)*
Authenticity – *the extent to which researchers faithfully show a range of different realities and convey the feeling and tone of lives as they are lived*	➤ *Include participant quotes to support researchers' interpretations to show results are grounded in the data rather than just viewpoints of the researchers*

Consider the work you have done so far regarding qualitative "scenario 2" in terms of constructing a question, a search strategy, understanding the features of phenomenological research by looking at a hypothetical study, where reflexivity could have been introduced, and understanding how the hypothetical data was collected and analysed. I have summarized those things in the following table before we move on to applying the qualitative quality criteria and the tools for critical appraisal.

Table 11.3 Summary of work done so far regarding the hypothetical "parents' perceptions" study

Children's nurse question:			
What are parents' perceptions of non-pharmacological interventions for managing their children's pain post-elective surgery?			

P	Parents		
E	Non-pharmacological interventions for their child		
O	Perception in relation to managing their children's pain post-elective surgery		
D	This is a "how does someone feel" type question requiring qualitative studies, usually ones that have interviewed participants, to answer it		

Sample search strategy answer:			
P #1 Parents OR Carers	I/E #2 Child AND Non-pharmacological interventions OR Play OR Distraction OR Controlled breathing OR Cognitive behaviour therapy OR Parental comforting	O #3 Experience in relation to managing children's pain post-elective surgery	D Qualitative

#1 **AND** #2 **AND** #3 would provide a basic search strategy for evidence on parents' perceptions in relation to management of children's pain post-elective surgery looking at appropriate research designs that consider "how does it feel".

Remember previously I asked you to imagine you have found a relevant **qualitative study** using your search strategy, and you are starting to look at the characteristics and underpinning philosophy of this qualitative research design.

Table 11.4 Basic steps in descriptive phenomenology applied to HYPOTHETICAL "scenario 2"

State the research purpose.	Explore parents' perceptions of non-pharmacological interventions for managing their children's pain post-elective surgery.
Decide the study design/ theoretical framework.	Use a phenomenological study and follow the steps associated with such an approach – "methodological coherence" (Richards & Morse, 2007).
Identify the participants of interest and select a sample. Describe the setting and the context.	After obtaining ethical approval to carry out the study, approach parents to explore their perceptions of non-pharmacological interventions for managing their children's pain post-elective surgery. Explain the purpose of the study, its benefits, risks, and the voluntary nature of taking part before obtaining their written informed consent. They needed to have experienced the phenomenon and be willing to talk about it in order to provide rich data. Provide characteristics of participants. Use pseudonyms to ensure the anonymity of participants. When asking parents to open up about a potentially upsetting experience, ensure support mechanisms are in place.
Collect data through semi-structured or unstructured in-depth interviews.	Conduct in-depth semi-structured interviews lasting 30–60 minutes in a quiet private space. Ask broad open questions to begin with such as "Please can you describe your experience of managing your child's pain after surgery?"., Be guided by the parents' answers to ask more probing questions. Make explicit what questions and prompts were used. Audio-record the interviews. Consider if more interviews with the same or different parents need to be carried out to reach data saturation.
Analyse narrative using a qualitative framework (Colaizzi, 1978, Wirihana et al, 2018).	Carefully listen to and transcribe verbatim each interview after each session. Also refer to any field notes or notes of non-verbal expression to aid interpretations. Return the transcripts to parents to check it reflects what they said. Then read multiple times. Highlight "stand out" phrases that seem to be key to indicate the experience of caring in these circumstances. Formulate meanings from these and put together into theme clusters and themes. Stop when no new themes emerge from the collected data. Develop an exhaustive description of the essence of the experience. Obtain feedback from parents regarding researchers' interpretations so they can say if their own perceptions are represented.

(Continued)

Table 11.4 (Continued)

Report on what has been discovered about these people's reality of this situation.	Let's imagine analysis of the data identified three major thematic areas which described parents' perceptions of non-pharmacological interventions for managing their children's pain post-elective surgery as feeling supported by professionals, familiarity with non-pharmacological interventions, and barriers to the use of non-pharmacological interventions. Present these with relevant quotes. After exploring the parents' perceptions, compare the results of the research study with other research literature.

Table 11.5 Qualitative quality criteria applied to qualitative "scenario 2"

QUALITATIVE Quality criteria (Lincoln & Guba, 1985), Guba and Lincoln (1994) applied to hypothetical scenario 2.	See if you can spot steps taken in the hypothetical scenario 2 to meet the qualitative quality criteria. Have a go before looking.
Confirmability – extent to which findings are based on study's participants and settings instead of researchers' biases	➤ *Didn't describe keeping a diary noting own role and motivations, so didn't appear in that respect to show reflexivity* ➤ *Appeared to have **audit trail**, but not **peer debriefing** and included participants' quotes to support researchers' interpretations to show results are grounded in the data rather than just viewpoints of the researchers*
Credibility – extent to which study's findings are believable to others	➤ *Used some **multiple data sources*** ➤ *Data triangulation – used transcripts and field notes* ➤ *Theory triangulation – compared to someone else's theory on this topic* ➤ ***Prolonged engagement or persistent observation** – said 30- to 60-minute interviews and re-interviewed in some instances* ➤ ***Respondent validation** of interview transcripts and themes was sought*

(Continued)

Table 11.5 (Continued)

Dependability – extent to which findings are consistent in relation to the context in which they were generated.	➤ *Did state* **member checks** *were done to check researcher reporting precisely what people say* ➤ *Did state collected data until no new data emerged* (**saturation**) ➤ *Did state carried out detailed audit trail documenting changes* ➤ *Direct quotes*
Transferability – extent to which findings can be transferred/applied in other settings	➤ **Thick descriptions** – *stated they collected information on population characteristics and context, but sampling strategy needs to be clearer*
Authenticity – the extent to which researchers faithfully show a range of different realities and convey the feeling and tone of lives as they are lived	➤ *Did state used direct quotes*

I mentioned in chapters on quantitative research that formal reporting guidelines have been developed for randomised controlled trials (CONSORT) and non-randomised observational studies (STROBE) to improve the quality of reporting these study types.

The Consolidated Criteria for Reporting Qualitative Research (COREQ) (Tong et al, 2007) checklist was developed to improve reporting of **qualitative** studies (using interviews and focus groups) (Tong et al, 2007). The Standards for Reporting Qualitative Research (SRQR) was developed later to provide clear standards of reporting **all** types of qualitative research (O'Brien et al, 2014).

The CASP tool for qualitative studies is a widely taught tool used to appraise qualitative studies that looks at study quality. You will recognise features in both the checklists and the appraisal tool that we have already discussed in this and the previous chapter, and again you will see your hard work is paying off.

Box 11.1   Features the COREQ document states it is important to clearly describe

The personal characteristics of the researcher – Could they have influenced the researchers' observations and interpretations?

The relationship of the researcher with participants – Could it have impacted on the participants' responses and on their own understanding of the phenomena?

Remember we talked about being reflexive earlier?

The theoretical framework underpinning their study e.g. phenomenology/ethnography/grounded theory – Did the researchers follow it?

Remember we talked about methodological coherence?

The participants and context of the setting – Was there sufficient coverage of differing viewpoints? Might the context have affected how participants responded?

The questions and prompts used in data collection – What was the researcher's focus? Were participants encouraged to express their views?

Whether participants were recruited until no new relevant knowledge was obtained from new participants – Did they achieve data saturation?

Whether the use of multiple coders or other methods of researcher triangulation were used

If respondent validation was carried out – How do you know that the participants' own meanings and perspectives are represented and not restricted by the researchers' own motivations and knowledge?

If supporting quotations are provided

If findings, interpretations, and theories generated are clearly presented

Remember we talked about steps researchers could take to enhance confirmability, credibility, dependability, transferability, and authenticity of data?

The Critical Appraisal Skills Programme (CASP) tool for qualitative studies

This is a widely taught tool used to appraise qualitative studies that looks at study quality (the CASP tool for qualitative studies, 2018). My students often use this tool when appraising qualitative studies in their background literature for their assignments. Flemming and Noyes (2021) say that "a set of domains has been recommended that have evolved from extensive practice (rather than empirical study)" regarding considering methodological limitations of such studies, and the CASP tool for qualitative studies maps onto these domains (Noyes et al, 2018).

Applying the CASP tool for qualitative studies to our parents' perceptions study

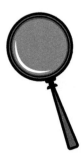

The CASP tool for qualitative research asks things like whether the study had clearly focused aims and whether a qualitative approach was appropriate, so being able to say what the PEO was helps determine if it asks a clearly focused question, and identifying that the research seeks to interpret the subjective experiences of research participants helps to determine if it was a qualitative study.

Once it has been established that it is a qualitative study, more detailed questions follow regarding the design, so explaining why phenomenology was appropriate to explore parents' perceptions in relation to managing their children's' pain with non-pharmacological interventions post-elective surgery.

Then questions about the sampling and data collection strategy follow. Who, how, and why the sample was chosen. If interviews were carried out, was an interview schedule used, where were they carried out, were they transcribed and recorded, did they continue until data saturation was reached? Regarding reflexivity, had the relationship between researcher and participants been adequately considered?

For example, was the researcher also the care provider? Was it clear if the researcher critically examined their own role, potential bias, and influence during each stage of the research process? Did they keep a diary, and was there an audit trail?

Then questions regarding data analysis follow, such as if there is an in-depth description of the analysis process. If thematic analysis is used, is it clear how the categories/themes were derived from the data? If sufficient data are presented to support the findings, did the researcher use participant quotes and carry out prolonged engagement, such as the length of time the interview took or going back to do a second interview? To what extent are contradictory data taken into account? Did they go back to the participants (respondent validation) and fellow researchers (peer debriefing) to check their interpretations of the data?

Are the findings clearly stated with questions relating to credibility (e.g. having more than one analyst, having interviews and field notes). Does the researcher discuss the contribution the study makes to existing knowledge or understanding? Have the researchers discussed transferability – whether or how the findings can be transferred to other populations – and have they provided "thick" descriptions of context and participant characteristics?

How can you use this in assignments?

I said earlier students are often asked to be critical rather than purely descriptive in their assignments, thus making a judgement about the trustworthiness of the research. Let's apply the CASP tool for qualitative studies to our hypothetical qualitative study looking at parents' perceptions of non-pharmacological interventions for managing their children's pain post-elective surgery, which found three major thematic areas: feeling supported by professionals, familiarity with non-pharmacological interventions, and barriers to the use of non-pharmacological interventions. Do you believe their data? In this hypothetical study there was nothing noted about keeping a diary describing the researcher's own role and motivations, so it didn't appear in that respect to show reflexivity. It appeared to have an audit trail, but no peer debriefing and included participants' quotes to support researchers' interpretations to show results are grounded in the data rather than just viewpoints of the researchers. It used some multiple data sources e.g. data triangulation – used transcripts and field notes – and theory triangulation – as it was compared to someone else's theory on this topic. Prolonged engagement was present – it said 30- to 60-minute interviews were carried out and parents re-interviewed in some instances. There was respondent validation of interview transcripts and themes. The researcher also stated data was collected until no new data emerged (saturation). No sampling strategy was provided, and it lacked "thick" descriptions – so the study lacked context and population characteristics that would have made findings meaningful to others. So would you trust this study? Would it enrich your practice? Including paragraphs like this in your work would get you points for demonstrating critical thinking.

Summary

- Critical appraisal is the process of carefully and systematically examining research to judge its trustworthiness and its value and relevance in a particular context (Burls, 2009).
- The COREQ and SQRQ statements are useful to inform you WHAT should be included in a qualitative study and give their reasons WHY.
- You have already learned that a phenomenological study is a research approach designed to answer a **"how does it feel"** question.
- Ask yourself: is it confirmable – are findings are based on the study's participants and settings instead of researchers' biases – look for reflexivity of the researcher, for example.
- Is it credible and believable to others – look for respondent validation, for example.

- Is it dependable – findings are consistent in relation to the context in which they were generated; look for an audit trail, for example.
- Is it transferable – findings can be transferred/applied in other settings – look for thick descriptions of participant characteristics and settings.
- Is it authentic – were there quotes that conveyed the lived experience?
- In this chapter we have considered the CASP tool for appraisal of qualitative studies and applied it to our hypothetical parents' perceptions of non-pharmacological interventions for their children's pain post-surgery.
- Flemming and Noyes (2021) say that a set of domains has been recommended that have evolved from extensive practice (rather than empirical study) that should be considered when assessing methodological limitations of a qualitative study, and the CASP tool for qualitative studies maps onto these domains (Flemming & Noyes, 2021).

References

Burls A. (2009) *What is Critical Appraisal?* The Bandolier Report. http://www.bandolier.org.uk/painres/download/whatis/What_is_critical_appraisal.pdf?msclkid=2ee70a20bdfe11ecaff1d5d9317b676b

Colaizzi P. (1978) Psychological research as the phenomenologist views it. In Vale RS, King M (Eds) *Existential-Phenomenological Alternatives for Psychology*. New York NY: Oxford University Press.

Critical Appraisal Skills Programme. (2018) *CASP (Qualitative) Checklist*. https://casp-uk.b-cdn.net/wp-content/uploads/2018/03/CASP-Qualitative-Checklist-2018_fillable_form.pdf. Accessed on 12/10/2021.

Flemming K, Noyes J. (2021) Qualitative evidence synthesis: Where are we at? *International Journal of Qualitative Methods*. doi: 10.1177/1609406921993276

Guba E, Lincoln Y. (1994) Competing paradigms in qualitative research. In Denzin N, Lincoln Y (Eds) *Handbook of Qualitative Research* (pp. 105–117). Thousand Oaks, CA: Sage.

Lincoln YS, Guba EG. (1985) *Naturalistic Inquiry*. Beverly Hills, CA: Sage.

Noyes J, Booth A, Flemming K, Garside R, Harden A, Lewin S, Pantoja T, Hannes K, Cargo M, Thomas J. (2018) Cochrane qualitative and implementation methods group guidance paper 3: Methods for assessing methodological limitations, data extraction and synthesis, and confidence in synthesized qualitative findings. *Journal of Clinical Epidemiology*; 97: 49–58. doi: 10.1016/j.jclinepi.2017.06.020

O'Brien BC, Harris IB, Beckman TJ, Reed DA, Cook DA. (2014) Standards for reporting qualitative research: a synthesis of recommendations. *Academic Medicine*; 89(9), September. doi: 10.1097/ACM.0000000000000388 CTDC

Polit DF, Beck CT. (2018) *Essentials of Nursing Research: Appraising Evidence for Nursing Practice*. 9th edn. Philadelphia. Wolters Kluwer.

Richards L, Morse JM. (2007) *Readme First for a User's Guide to Qualitative Methods*. Thousand Oaks: Sage Publications.

Tong A, Sainsbury P, Craig J. (2007) Consolidated criteria for reporting qualitative research (COREQ): A 32-item checklist for interviews and focus groups. *International Journal for Quality in Health Care*; 19(6): 349–357.

Walsh D, Downe S. (2006) Appraising the quality of qualitative research. *Midwifery*; 22(2): 108–119. ISSN 0266-6138. doi: 10.1016/j.midw.2005.05.004. (www.sciencedirect.com/science/article/pii/S0266613805000586) discusses common quality things looked for.

Wirihana L, Welch A, Williamson M, Christensen M, Bakon S, Craft J. (2018) Using Colaizzi's method of data analysis to explore the experiences of nurse academics teaching on satellite campuses. *Nurse Research*; 16; 25(4): 30–34. doi: 10.7748/nr.2018.e1516. PMID: 29546965

Step 4

Make a decision to implement the evidence

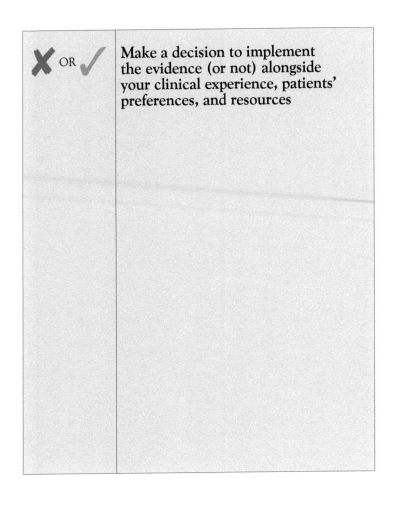

Make a decision to implement the evidence (or not) alongside your clinical experience, patients' preferences, and resources

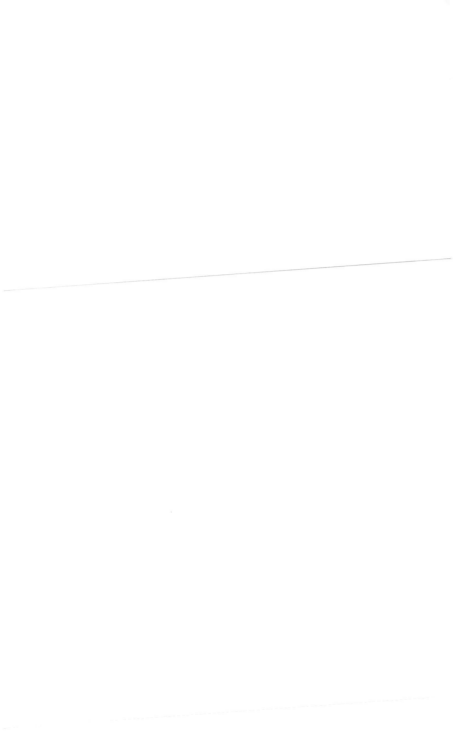

12 Why we need systematic reviews and initiatives like the Cochrane Library

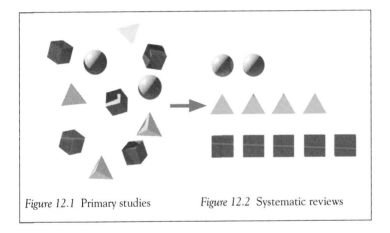

Figure 12.1 Primary studies   *Figure 12.2* Systematic reviews

Do you think it is it possible to find, appraise, and synthesise all the primary quantitative and qualitative studies to keep on top of the evidence about **"what works best"** and **"how it makes people feel"**?

Imagine you have come up with your research question, searched for evidence, found a primary piece of research, and critically appraised it using an appropriate appraisal tool and interpreted the results – ALL THE WORK SO FAR IN THIS BOOK! But then you find there are lots more primary studies that have tried to answer your question!

You are a busy health care professional – you understand that you need to refer to the evidence and research to inform your decisions,

DOI: 10.4324/9781003156017-16

but do you have time to find, appraise, and synthesise all these findings? Would you have the complete picture if you didn't? What if you found one poor-quality study that said something worked but there were ten other better-quality studies with less bias that said the intervention didn't work – how could that impact on your practice?

Luckily for us all, there are systematic reviews and collaborations that produce them such as the Cochrane Collaboration, the EPPI-centre, and the Joanna Briggs Institute – and it is this type of **secondary** research and such groups that we will consider in this chapter. Remember that with primary research the researcher "goes out" and conducts the research. In secondary research, the researcher systematically reviews OTHER PEOPLE'S primary research, but needs to employ the same rigour to ensure the systematic reviews produced are also trustworthy.

A systematic review is prepared using a systematic approach. Each of the steps, such as the process of constructing a PICO/PEO, the process of constructing a search strategy, the process of appraising the included studies, and the process of extracting and synthesising the data, are all described in detail and made transparent in a systematic review (this is absent from a traditional literature review). Sounding familiar?

Quantitative systematic reviews and meta-analysis

Quantitative systematic reviews and meta-analysis are techniques for pooling **quantitative** research evidence (usually RCTs) on the effectiveness of a health care therapy or intervention (Chalmers et al, 2002, Mulrow, 1994, Nagendrababu et al, 2020).

Remember in the first chapter I said if we want to know "what works best", at the top of the hierarchy of evidence would be systematic reviews of RCTs.

Even better than this would be a meta-analysis, which is a type of systematic review that involves the synthesis of results/effect measures from several RCTs to yield an **overall** effect measure and confidence interval. The RCTs have to be very similar to do this.

A narrative synthesis is done when a meta-analysis can't be done, e.g. if the included RCTs are clinically diverse or they are at risk of bias, then individual study results only are presented and discussed.

Box 12.1   Some milestones in relation to quantitative systematic reviews (cited by Chalmers et al, 2002 and Clarke, 2015)

- Back in the 18th century James Lind wrote about the difficulty of synthesising information and was quoted as saying, "Before the subject could be set in a clear and proper light it was necessary to remove a great deal of rubbish".
- Archie Cochrane 1972 is often quoted as saying, "It is surely a great criticism of our profession we have not organised a critical summary, by speciality or sub-speciality, adapted periodically, of all relevant randomised controlled trials".
- Chalmers (1978) and his team systematically reviewed evidence for interventions related to pregnancy and childbirth.
- Sackett in 1989 published work on critically appraising research and coined the term "scientific medicine", which was later changed to EBM and which he defined as "the conscientious, explicit and judicious use of current best evidence in making decisions about the care of individual patients".
- In 1992 the Cochrane Collaboration was established to organise individuals to produce systematic reviews establishing the effectiveness (or not) of health care interventions.
- Then came the Campbell Collaboration, which was established for the effectiveness of social interventions and broader public policy.
- The Evidence for Policy and Practice information and coordination centre (EPPI-centre) was established, which was interested in evaluations of interventions in education and social welfare.

> ## Box 12.2   Purposes quantitative systematic reviews can serve (Mulrow, 1994)
>
> - Can tell you what works best
> - Can highlight what doesn't work or does harm
> - Can avoid unnecessary primary research
>   If, for example, there was clear evidence that some intervention worked after the fifth trial, there would be no need to conduct a sixth trial.
> - Can provide new evidence
>   For example, show if some intervention was time or dose dependent
> - Can drive the research agenda
>   For example, by highlighting a lack of trials or good-quality trials

Consideration of a hypothetical quantitative SR

So let us consider our "what works best" question regarding honey for oral mucositis. In the previous chapters we considered, in our quest to be an EBP practitioner, finding a relevant hypothetical RCT, after constructing a suitable PICO, then searching, appraising, and extracting the results.

Following our critical appraisal exercise we decided it was not at risk of selection bias, detection bias, or attrition bias – but it was at risk of performance bias. We also saw in this hypothetical study that the results for people having oral mucositis after 1 week were given as a risk ratio of 0.8 with a 95% confidence interval of 0.7 to 0.9. This was a statistically significant result for this hypothetical trial, suggesting honey reduces the presence of oral mucositis when compared with saline at 1 week.

Let's now imagine a team of systematic reviewers are interested in effective interventions for radiation-induced oral mucositis and have found three RCTs, including our hypothetical trial (that we shall refer to as study 1 in our hypothetical SR), that have focused on honey vs. saline.

Three RCTs are better than one RCT in terms of informing the evidence base and decision making, I think you can agree? Remember with 95% confidence intervals it is like saying if you drew 100 samples at random, 95% of the samples would contain the population parameter. With one sample, you take the risk 5% of the time that you might not have the true result. Therefore it is better to have lots of samples (so lots of RCTs).

In terms of presenting this info in the SR, the team would extract the PICO from each of the three trials to see if it fulfilled the scope of their SR (so their PICO). If it did, it would be an "included" study and would be critically appraised using the Cochrane Risk of Bias (ROB) tool. **You are already familiar with PICO and appraisal using the Cochrane ROB tool, right,** so don't be fazed if you see this in a quantitative SR. The Cochrane ROB tool focuses solely on sources of bias because Cochrane argued that this is preferential when systematically reviewing trials of effectiveness, as bias impacts on the internal validity of the study (Higgins et al, 2011). Remember internal validity is the ability of the study to show X causes Y – so you don't want any other systematic variation between the two groups apart from the intervention.

The reviewers would do this with the two remaining honey studies to be included in the systematic review (let's call them study 2 and study 3) so the reader could see how they fulfilled the systematic reviewer's **PICO** and **ROB** in these studies. I want you to see that you are familiar with all of these processes.

Table 12.1 What the systematic reviewers would do with included studies

Study 1	Study 2	Study 3
PICO extracted	PICO extracted	PICO extracted
ROB assessment made	ROB assessment made	ROB assessment made

As well as critically appraising the included studies, the systematic reviewers would extract the results of all three included trials to see if honey was having an effect.

Remember the results from our **hypothetical** honey trial for the presence or absence of oral mucositis (study 1 in the hypothetical SR).

Box 12.3 Included study 1

The RR was 0.8, which is less than 1, so that tells us that events (presence of oral mucositis after 1 week) are happening less in the experimental I/(honey) group than in the control (C/saline) group.

Remember the 95% confidence interval for this hypothetical data was 0.7 to 0.9. Because the 95% confidence interval did NOT include the "no difference" RR result of 1 in the confidence interval range, this **would** be considered a statistically significant answer – remember, though, this is a hypothetical example!

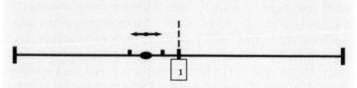

Figure 12.3 Number line to show RR = 0.8 95% CI 0.7 to 0.9

Let's imagine the following results from the three included studies in the **hypothetical** SR.

Table 12.2 Results from the three included studies in the hypothetical systematic review

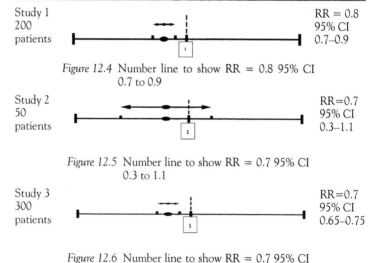

Study 1
200
patients

RR = 0.8
95% CI
0.7–0.9

Figure 12.4 Number line to show RR = 0.8 95% CI
0.7 to 0.9

Study 2
50
patients

RR=0.7
95% CI
0.3–1.1

Figure 12.5 Number line to show RR = 0.7 95% CI
0.3 to 1.1

Study 3
300
patients

RR=0.7
95% CI
0.65–0.75

Figure 12.6 Number line to show RR = 0.7 95% CI
0.65 to 0.75

If the three trials were very similar in terms of PICO and how the outcomes were measured, it might be possible to do a meta-analysis, so as well as three separate risk ratios and confidence intervals, an **overall effect measure (in this case, an overall risk ratio and confidence interval)** could be calculated. A quick way to check for similarity is to look at the confidence intervals for each study – if they don't overlap, the studies are likely to be different. More rigorous tests of similarity include statistical testing (Sedgwick, 2015).

Table 12.3 Hypothetical forest plot to indicate how it might appear in a systematic review: comparison: honey vs. saline, outcome 1: mucositis (any) – so a dichotomous outcome

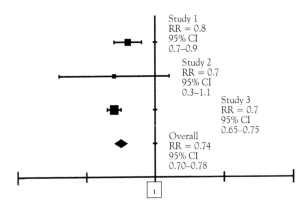

Figure 12.7 Forest plot

Forest plots are the usual way to show results of individual studies and meta-analyses in quantitative systematic reviews (Lalkhen & McCluskey, 2008, Nagendrababu et al, 2020, Sedgwick, 2015). It helps you, the busy health care professional, see in a visual way if the intervention of interest (in this case, honey) has had a statistically significant effect or not when **all** the included studies (those that fulfil the PICO and three in our hypothetical example) have been taken into account. The largest trial would carry more weight, as it would be expected to provide the most precise estimate (indicated by a bigger "blob" and narrower confidence intervals – see study 3). The overall effect measure is conveyed by the diamond – the centre being the **point estimate** and the outer reaches indicating the **95% confidence interval**.

It appears in this **hypothetical** forest plot that honey has had a significant effect, as the overall effect measure does not include the "no difference" result of 1 for this dichotomous outcome.

I have simplified the explanation of the forest plot for you to get the basic idea and to encourage you to read up more on what is involved in their construction and interpretation (Lalkhen & McCluskey, 2008, Nagendrababu et al, 2020).

Another very important consideration is that quantitative systematic reviewers don't just extract and synthesise the results and conclude whether the intervention of interest worked or not. This has to be tempered with the quality of the included studies. The three honey trials in our example may have fulfilled the PICO, but what if following appraisal, they were all found to have a lot of bias? Remember in Chapters 7 and 8 we discussed that any interpretation of results **must** be influenced by how biased or unbiased the RCTs were. An observed difference could be due to this bias (systematic differences in the way the groups were treated) rather than chance or the intervention of interest. This in turn will influence the recommendations of the systematic reviewers for practice and for further research.

Have a look at the abstract of a quantitative systematic review – you will often see the effect measures within it. Can you interpret them? Within the SR you can view the forest plots and practice interpreting them (tip: remember for dichotomous data – the "no difference"/null result is 1; look to see if the RR, OR, or CI range includes this value, and for continuous data – the "no difference"/null result is 0; check to see if the MD or CI range includes this value).

The Cochrane Collaboration

This group takes its name from Archie Cochrane (mentioned earlier). Following on from the pregnancy and childbirth group's work in Oxford in the 1980s, the Cochrane Collaboration was formed, with the UK Cochrane Centre (1992) being one of the first such centres.

This collaboration recognised the need in the early 1990s for primary research (predominantly RCTs) to be systematically reviewed regularly to aid decision making about "what works best" in health care and set about organising individuals to produce SRs of effectiveness of health care interventions. The collaboration has grown into an international group, with contributors to SR production worldwide. If you look on their website they have special collections of SRs rapidly put together to help countries when they have faced a disaster causing a health crisis such as earthquakes, tsunamis, and pandemics, to access effective evidence-based interventions, e.g. to rehydrate and to treat crush fractures, head injuries, diarrhoea, sepsis, post-traumatic stress, and viral infections.

Think of the many interventions you use, recommend, advise against, and wonder if they work or even do harm – the Cochrane Library is the electronic home of Cochrane systematic reviews looking at the effectiveness of health care interventions. This should be one of the first places you look to find high-level evidence for if a health care intervention works or not. Remember the hierarchy of evidence discussed in the first chapter, with SRs of RCTs at the top for "what works best"? SRs are essentially dynamic documents, as they should be regularly updated as new trial data becomes available. Remember hypotheses are rejected or not rejected and the "truth" might change in light of new findings.

Information from such SRs are not clinical guidelines, although they are used to inform them (see the next chapter) and aren't meant to be universally prescriptive. Remember in Chapter 1 we discussed clinical decision making does not only rely on evidence, but on clinical experience, patient preferences, and resources. What if the evidence for larval therapy was strong regarding how effective it was at debriding wounds but a patient said they didn't want it? The SR of RCTs might be there, but it is against the patient's personal preference. This is where qualitative SRs or qualitative research could be useful to enrich our understanding of patients' preferences (Booth, 2017).

With these field examples, have a look on Cochrane Library to see if there are any quantitative SRs of effectiveness on them (tip: use a PICO framework to construct a search strategy).

Table 12.4 Questions from the different fields of nursing regarding "what works best"

Adult field example: Does **topical negative pressure** heal chronic wounds?	Child field example: Does **emollient cream** resolve childhood eczema?
Mental health field example: Do **coping strategies** reduce stress in carers of relatives with dementia?	Learning disabilities field example: Does **exercise** reduce anxiety in people with a learning disability?

Qualitative systematic reviews

Qualitative systematic reviews are techniques for pooling qualitative research to analyse human experience and cultural and social phenomena. The methods for conducting these are still evolving.

Box 12.4   Milestones in relation to qualitative systematic reviews

- Noblit and Hare (1988) were instrumental in the area of synthesising qualitative data. They describe such reviews as aggregated or as interpretative. The aggregated review summarises the data; interpretative approaches, as the name suggests, interpret the data, and from that interpretation, "new understandings may develop" – referred to as *meta-ethnography*.
- Sandelowski and Barroso (2007) discussed "enhancing the utility of qualitative research".
- Popay et al (1998) produced the "Rationale and standards for the systematic review of qualitative literature in health services research".
- Joanna Briggs Institute (Adelaide) (1990s) – Set up to develop methodologies and guidance on the process of systematic reviews. Focused on meta-aggregation of primary research findings to inform policy and practice.
- Cochrane Collaboration – Cochrane Qualitative and Implementation Methods Group (CQRMG) in 2006 coined the term qualitative evidence synthesis (QES) (Noyes et al, 2008).

> ### Box 12.5   Purposes qualitative systematic reviews may serve
>
> - When wishing to assess meaningfulness, appropriateness, acceptability, and/or feasibility of an intervention or practice
> - Needs and priorities of users of health and social care
> - Pooling research evidence on people's experiences
> - Going beyond the context of the original studies (Noblit & Hare, 1988)

Consideration of a hypothetical qualitative systematic review

So let us consider briefly our "how does it feel" question regarding parents' perceptions of non-pharmacological interventions to manage their child's pain post-elective surgery. In the previous chapters we considered, in our quest to be an EBP practitioner, we found a relevant hypothetical phenomenological study and after constructing a suitable PEO, searched, then appraised, and extracted the results.

Following our critical appraisal exercise, we decided some steps had been taken to improve the confirmability, credibility, dependability, and transferability of the study, but it lacked some reflexivity and peer debriefing. We also saw this hypothetical study generated three themes – feeling supported by professionals, familiarity with non-pharmacological interventions, and barriers to the use of non-pharmacological interventions

Let's now imagine a group of systematic reviewers are interested in parents' **perceptions** of non-pharmacological interventions to manage their child's pain. They might find different qualitative studies besides our phenomenological study that have different philosophical underpinnings and data collection and analysis approaches that go with, say, interpretive phenomenology or grounded theory. These studies may have generated similar or different themes. They may have described experiences or interpreted them.

It is beyond the scope of this book to go into how qualitative research could be systematically reviewed, but suffice it to say there are ongoing debates about how best to do this. The term qualitative evidence synthesis (QES) is the preferred term of the Cochrane Qualitative and Implementation Methods Group (Booth, 2016, Noyes et al, 2008). Booth says it acknowledges that qualitative research requires its own methods for synthesis, which reflects the nature of the qualitative paradigm, rather than simply using the same methods devised for systematic reviews of quantitative research (Booth, 2016).

With these field examples have a look at Cochrane/JBI to see if there are any qualitative SRs to provide descriptions, insights, and understanding of the impact of these experiences on people (tip: use the PIO/PEO framework to construct a search strategy).

Table 12.5 Questions from the different fields of nursing regarding "how someone feels"

Adult field example: What is the impact of a non-healing venous leg ulcer in adults?	Child field example: What is the impact of repeated surgeries in children?
Mental health field example: What is the impact of repeated miscarriages in women?	Learning disabilities field example: What is the impact on family carers for a child with profound multiple learning disabilities?

Steps in SR process

As a lone health care professional, if you have a research question about "what works best" or "how does it make someone feel", you may search, appraise, and synthesise the results from one or two primary studies. You now understand hopefully what the SR reviewer does – the same processes you have learned about but on a larger, more comprehensive, transparent scale looking extensively for the research on that topic, unpublished as well as published research, English and non-English research, with another reviewer involved in selecting, appraising, extracting, and synthesising the data to reduce bias. This saves you, the busy health care professional, an enormous amount of time! Similar processes are followed by both a quantitative and qualitative systematic reviewer, but the comprehensiveness of the search differs, as do the types of studies included and subsequent approaches to appraisal, analysis, and synthesis, with data either being quantitative (e.g. to see the effectiveness/exposure to something) or qualitative (e.g. to see the impact of something on the individual in terms of feelings/experiences). Look at Table 12.6 to see the similarities between the EBP processes (which you are familiar with) and SR processes.

Table 12.6 Similarities between the EBP processes and SR processes

Steps	EBP process	SR process
PICOD PICO PEO	1. Pose a focused research question	1. **Define an appropriate therapeutic** question (PICOD/ PEO)
	2. Search for the evidence	2. Search the literature: Electronically and manually Published and unpublished English and non- English
	3. Critically appraise the evidence	3. Assess the studies for eligibility (see if PICO/PEO fulfilled) For included studies, assess quality (using appropriate critical appraisal tools) Extract data and report findings (expressed as e.g. risk ratios/odds ratios and confidence intervals or mean differences and confidence intervals for quantitative studies or e.g. aggregated or interpreted themes for qualitative studies)
X OR ✓	4. Make a decision to implement the evidence (or not) alongside your clinical experience, patients' preferences, and resources	4. In a quantitative SR summarise the evidence in "evidence tables"; compare the benefits and harms Make a decision to implement the evidence (or not) alongside your clinical experience, patients' preferences (potentially informed by QES), and resources
	5. Evaluate this	5. Evaluate this

Just as you learned how to critically appraise primary quantitative and qualitative studies, you should critically appraise secondary research/SRs, as they could also have limitations, e.g. the processes were not carried out fully or transparently, or with one reviewer only, or with inappropriate aggregation of studies, or recommendations are not based firmly on the quality of the evidence presented, for example (Liberati et al, 2009).

In the late 1990s the Quality of Reporting of Meta-analysis (QUOROM) statement was produced, which evolved into the Preferred Reporting Items for SRs and Meta-analyses (PRISMA) statement (Liberati et al, 2009) which was developed to improve the reporting of quantitative SRs.

CASP also has a tool to appraise SRs (CASP, 2018). The Grading of Recommendations, Assessment, Development and Evaluations (GRADE) approach provides guidance for assessing how much confidence to place in findings from systematic reviews of quantitative research – so how certain review authors are that an effect measure (from several samples/RCTs) represents the true population effect (Balshem et al, 2011). Remember in Chapter 9 when assessing primary quantitative studies for risk of bias, it needs to be done for each outcome or result, as bias can impact differently on different outcomes. A GRADE assessment is also applied to each review **outcome**, which includes the risk of bias in the included studies, the relevance or directness of these studies to the review question, the consistency of results from these studies, the precision of the estimate, and the risk of publication bias in the contributing evidence (Balshem et al, 2011).

The Confidence in the Evidence from Reviews of Qualitative Research (GRADE-CERQual) approach provides guidance for assessing how much confidence to place in findings from systematic reviews of qualitative research (or qualitative evidence syntheses) (Lewin et al, 2015).

Summary

- In the chapters so far, we have considered how to try to be an EB practitioner by putting a good research question together, constructing a search strategy, and appraising and interpreting primary quantitative or qualitative research found and making a judgement about if it can reliably inform one's practice.

- You have experienced first-hand in this book that judging a piece of research for its trustworthiness and interpreting its findings is an involved process.

- It would be impossible for the busy health care professional to keep on top of this primary research, which is being produced all the time.

- Luckily for us, initiatives have developed secondary research approaches – predominantly systematic reviews. This is when primary research carried out by others is rigorously searched for and appraised and relevant data extracted and synthesised to answer pertinent research questions – all the processes you have learned about so far!

- With quantitative systematic reviews, great care is taken to find all relevant studies, to appraise each included study, to extract and synthesise results from included studies, and to present a summary of the findings, having considered any methodological flaws and using more than one reviewer for each of the processes.

- Cochrane's quantitative systematic reviews largely focus on RCTs and sometimes cohort studies to look at the effectiveness of health care interventions. Cochrane's sister organisation, Campbell, largely focuses on the effectiveness of social care interventions. The EPPI-centre focuses on educational and social care interventions.

- With qualitative systematic reviews, the extent of searching is driven by the need to reach theoretical saturation, there are debates for and against critical appraisal in QES, and data synthesis can be an aggregative or interpretive process (Noyes et al, 2008).

- Joanna Briggs Institute, which has relatively recently joined forces with Cochrane, produces qualitative systematic reviews of qualitative studies to look at the impact of/exposure to some health care issue.

- Quantitative systematic review methodology is more developed than qualitative systematic review methodology, with the latter referred to by some as QES.

- So hopefully you can start to appreciate how primary studies inform SRs but critical appraisal of SRs is still necessary.

References

Balshem H, Helfand M, Schunemann HJ, Oxman AD, Kunz R, Brozek J. et al. (2011) GRADE guidelines: 3. Rating the quality of evidence. *Journal of Clinical Epidemiology*; 64: 401–406.

Booth A. (2016) Searching for qualitative research for inclusion in systematic reviews: a structured methodological review. *Systematic Reviews*; 5(1): 74. doi: 10.1186/s13643-016-0249-x

Booth A. (2017) Qualitative evidence synthesis. In Facey K, Ploug Hansen H, Single A (Eds) *Patient Involvement in Health Technology Assessment* (pp. 187–199). Singapore: Adis. ISBN 9789811040689

Chalmers I, Hedges LV, Cooper H. (2002) A brief history of research synthesis. *Evaluation & the Health Professions*; 25(1): 12–37. doi: 10.1177/0163278702025001003

Clarke M. (2015) History of evidence synthesis to assess treatment effects: personal reflections on something that is very much alive. *JLL Bulletin: Commentaries on the History of Treatment Evaluation*. www.jameslindlibrary.org/articles/hist#ory-of-evidence-synthesis-to-assess-treatment-effects-personal-reflections-on-something-that-is-very-much-alive/

Cochrane AL. (1972) *Effectiveness and Efficiency: Random Reflections on Health Services*. London: Nuffield Provincial Hospitals Trust.

Critical Appraisal Skills Programme. (2018) *CASP Systematic Reviews Checklist*. https://casp-uk.b-cdn.net/wp-content/uploads/2018/03/CASP-Systematic-Review-Checklist-2018_fillable-form.pdf. Accessed on 03/11/2021.

Higgins JPT, Altman DG, Gotzsche PC, Juni P, Moher D, Oxman AD. et al. (2011) The Cochrane collaboration's tool for assessing risk of bias in randomised trials. *BMJ*; 343: d5928. doi: 10.1136/bmj.d5928

Lalkhen GA, McCluskey A. (2008) Statistics V: Introduction to clinical trials and systematic reviews. *Continuing Education in Anaesthesia Critical Care & Pain*; 8(4): 143–146. ISSN 1743-1816. doi: 10.1093/bjaceaccp/mkn023; www.sciencedirect.com/science/article/pii/S1743181617304754

Lewin S, Glenton C, Munthe-Kaas H, Carlsen B, Colvin CJ, Gülmezoglu M. et al. (2015) Using qualitative evidence in decision making for health and social interventions: An approach to assess confidence in findings from qualitative evidence syntheses (GRADE-CERQual). *PLoS Medicine*; 12(10): e1001895. doi: 10.1371/journal.pmed.1001895

Liberati A, Altman DG, Tetzlaff J. et al. (2009) The PRISMA statement for reporting systematic reviews and meta-analyses of studies that evaluate health care interventions: Explanation and elaboration. *PLoS Medicine*; 6: e1000100.

Mulrow C. (1994) Systematic reviews: Rationale for systematic reviews. *BMJ (Clinical Research Ed.)*; 309: 597–599. doi: 10.1136/bmj.309.6954.597.

Nagendrababu V, Dilokthornsakul P, Jinatongthai P, Veetil SK, Pulikkotil SJ, Duncan HF, Dummer PMH. (2020) Glossary for systematic reviews and meta-analyses. *International Endodontic Journal*; 53: 232–249.

Noblit G, Hare R. (1988) *Meta-ethnography: Synthesising Qualitative Studies* (Qualitative research methods, Series 11). Thousand Oaks, CA: SAGE.

Noyes J, Popay J, Pearson A, Hannes K, Booth A. (2008) Chapter 20: Qualitative research and Cochrane reviews. In Higgins JPT, Green S (Eds) *Cochrane Handbook for Systematic Reviews of Interventions*. Version 5.0.1 [updated September 2008]. The Cochrane Collaboration. http://handbook.cochrane.org/chapter_20/20_qualitative_research_and_cochrane_reviews.htm.

Popay J, Rogers A, Williams G. (1998) Rationale and standards for the systematic review of qualitative literature in health services research. *Qualitative Health Research*; 8: 341–351.

Sandelowski M, Barroso J. (2007) *Handbook for Synthesising Qualitative Research*. New York: Springer.

Sedgwick P. (2015) How to read a forest plot in a meta-analysis. *BMJ*; 351: h4028. doi: 10.1136/bmj.h4028.

13 Clinical guidelines and implementation of EBP

In this chapter you will see how it all comes together. If primary research can be pulled together into systematic reviews, which are then fed into clinical guidelines and implementation is supported, this would enable many more health care professionals to use best evidence to inform practice.

The alternative is that the evidence just "sits there" unused and practice continues to be based on tradition, authority, and expert opinion, which may result in effective treatments not being used or known about and ineffective or even harmful interventions and practices still being used.

You have seen how much work needs to go into producing primary research and secondary research (systematic reviews) to ensure they are trustworthy, and it is no different for the production of clinical guidelines, which we will consider in more detail in this chapter.

What is a clinical guideline?

"Practice guidelines that are evidence based, combining a synthesis and appraisal of research evidence with specific recommendations for clinical decisions" (Polit & Beck, 2018).

'Statements that include recommendations intended to optimise patient care that are informed by a systematic review of evidence and an assessment of the benefits and harms of alternative care options" (Graham et al, 2011).

"NICE guidelines provide care standards within the NHS for healthcare professionals, patients and their carers on the prevention,

DOI: 10.4324/9781003156017-17

treatment and care of people with specific diseases and conditions as well as recommendations on the organisation of services and social care" (National Guideline Centre, 2021).

What are the steps involved?

The steps for designing explicit, evidence-based guidelines were described in the late 1980s, and guess what – they involve formulating questions; searching the literature; appraising the evidence; summarising the evidence; and comparing the benefits, harms, and costs where possible in order to draw a conclusion about best practice.

Developing clinical guidelines

The National Institute for Health and Care Excellence (formerly the National Institute for Clinical Excellence; NICE), the UK government's guideline organisation, expect a rigorous methodology to be followed for clinical guideline production.

The National Guideline Centre (formerly the National Clinical Guideline Centre; NGC) develops evidence-based clinical guidelines on behalf of NICE. These guidelines are developed for the National Health Service (NHS) and establish recommendations on best practice.

Steps in clinical guideline development have been described by Hill et al (2011) and the National Guideline Centre (2021) and are detailed in guideline manuals and handbooks produced by NICE and the Scottish Intercollegiate Guideline Network (SIGN). I will outline them very briefly here so you can see you are already familiar with the processes involved.

- **1. Guideline topic is referred**
  Suggestions can come from lots of different sources and drivers. You can imagine that things like pandemics would be a strong driver, as would a disease that impacted on a lot of people. If some medication was very expensive, there might be a driver to look for other effective interventions that cost less. What if a cancer treatment was being offered in one post code but not another – a national guideline advising what was the best treatment might help reduce such inequalities and variations in practice.

- **2. Stakeholders register interest**
  A stakeholder is usually someone who has an interest or concern in something. Imagine a guideline being produced around interventions for dementia. Have a think for a moment who the stakeholders would be. Guideline producers have defined stakeholders as patient/carer organisations, national organisations that represent health care professionals, clinicians, companies that manufacture medicines/devices, providers and commissioners of health services, and statutory and research organisations (NICE, 2018, SIGN, 2011). Have a think how their interests might converge, diverge, or even compete. Health care professionals and clinicians might be most interested in what works best; patient/carer organisations might also be interested in what works best and also how it makes them feel. Companies that manufacture the medicines may have an interest in their drug/device being used to increase profit for their shareholders. Providers and commissioners of health services will have interest in if the interventions work and their costs. Research organisations may be interested in the research that has been done or still needs to be done.

- **3. Scope of guideline is prepared**
  Once the scope has been defined, the next stage is to produce focused clinical research questions which will help to identify the evidence needed from the subsequent systematic reviews. Guideline producers have stated that the types of clinical questions that may be asked can include epidemiology or aetiology of a disease; cost-effectiveness; accuracy of diagnostic tests; effectiveness of an intervention ("what works best" type questions); prognosis; clinical prediction models for diagnosis or prognosis; and experiences and views of patients, families, and service providers ("how does it feel" type questions) (NICE, 2018, Royal College of Paediatrics and Child Health, 2020). They say the exact number of clinical questions will depend on the extent of the scope and resources and recommend limiting them to up to about 15, incorporating economic evaluation if possible.

- **4. Guideline development group established**
  It is important for this group to be independent and to declare any conflicts of interest. Guideline producers say they usually comprise 10 to 12 members including health care professionals,

patient/carer representatives, professionals with expertise in the topic, technical experts in systematic reviewing, health economists, information scientists, and project managers who can carry out the work but represent the interests of the stakeholders (NICE, 2018, Royal College of Paediatrics and Child Health, 2020). The health care industry is not represented on guideline development groups (GDGs) because of potential conflicts of interest (NICE, 2018). It makes sense that steps need to be taken to ensure guidance is developed by independent and unbiased committees of experts – what if, for example, one of the members was a shareholder in a drug company who would benefit from, say, the prescribing of a certain drug? There is now a requirement that the GDGs have at least two lay members (Royal College of Paediatrics and Child Health, 2020). They work together for ~16 months, meeting every 4 to 6 weeks.

- **5. Draft guideline produced**
- **6. Final guideline produced**

The full clinical guideline must clearly show how the working group has moved from the evidence to the recommendation (Royal College of Paediatrics and Child Health, 2020). They are action based, and the recommendations can be strong or weak.

There are two ways to assess the quality of research studies: as a whole study or by outcome.

As a **whole study**. Evidence is categorised as levels 1, 2, 3, 4, or 5 depending on the type of study that is drawn from (e.g. systematic reviews, randomised control trials, cohort studies, cross-sectional studies, case-control studies, or case series) (Howick et al, 2011).

By **outcome**. If GRADE is used, the quality of systematic reviews is assessed and summarised by outcomes across all relevant studies and evidence is graded as high, moderate, low, or very low quality regarding the estimate of effect (remember risk ratios, odds ratios, mean differences, and confidence intervals and how bias may affect outcomes differently). If evidence was graded as high, this would suggest no further research is required, or if very low quality, much more research is required (Balshem et al, 2011). As well as considering risk of bias, GRADE takes into account imprecision, inconsistency, indirectness of study results, and publication bias (Balshem et al, 2011). Remember imprecise estimates can come from small studies, inconsistent results are indicated by studies whose confidence intervals don't overlap, and publication bias happens when studies that found a statistically significant difference are more likely to get published than studies that didn't.

- **7. Guideline implementation**
  Key recommendations are the recommendations likely to have the biggest impact on patient care and outcomes as a whole (Royal College of Paediatrics and Child Health, 2020).

  Clinical audit is a quality improvement process that involves measuring current practice against agreed standards. "Research is concerned with discovering the right thing to do; audit with ensuring that it is done right" (Smith, 1992, p. 905). This constitutes the final step of EBP, which is evaluation of the implementation of the evidence.

Use of quantitative research in clinical guidelines

Carroll (2017) reminds us that Sackett and colleagues, over 20 years ago, asserted that evidence-based practice involves the use of the "best external evidence" to inform clinical decision making. He also states that the evidence used to underpin clinical guidelines, including those produced by the NICE in the UK, is almost exclusively quantitative (Carroll, 2017). This makes sense, as the principal focus is efficacy and safety: the aim is to establish "what works". This is why as a nurse it is important to understand quantitative primary research approaches and quantitative systematic reviews.

Cochrane have recently announced they are signing a collaboration licence agreement with NICE. Cochrane has a long-established relationship with the NHS and the National Institute for Health Research (NIHR), and Cochrane reviews are already used to inform NICE guidelines. They said the agreement seeks to make this sharing of Cochrane evidence for use in NICE guidelines easier and more efficient.

Use of qualitative research in clinical guidelines

Glenton et al (2016) and Lewin and Glenton (2018) discuss how, in their work with the World Health Organization (WHO), they have explored ways of broadening the types of evidence used to develop evidence-informed guidance for health systems such as qualitative evidence syntheses (QES) (Booth et al 2017) to inform the values, acceptability, equity, and feasibility implications of its recommendations.

Carroll (2017) states that Sackett and colleagues were also clear that clinical practice should take account of patients' preferences, which is currently achieved by patient involvement in the process and by using primary qualitative research. He states, "The synthesis of several relevant qualitative studies can offer multiple perspectives as well as providing evidence of contradictory viewpoints that might otherwise be missed when considering a single study alone". So for patient preferences, which relates to "how someone feels", he advocates that an SR or QES of qualitative studies might be more informative (Carroll, 2017).

Consideration of how a hypothetical honey trial could be included in a hypothetical SR which is then included in a hypothetical clinical guideline

You have considered in a hypothetical scenario how a primary RCT might seek to answer the "what works best" question in relation to honey vs. saline on oral mucositis and how it might be included in a quantitative SR looking at interventions for oral mucositis. Have a think what clinical guideline it might appear in, e.g. something like "managing side effects of cancer treatments". Here I am trying to illustrate how primary research (RCTs) inform secondary research (SRs), which inform clinical guidelines.

Consideration of how a hypothetical parents' perceptions phenomenological study could be included in a hypothetical SR which is then included in a hypothetical clinical guideline

You have considered in a hypothetical scenario how a primary phenomenological study seeks to explore a "how does it feel" question in relation to parents' perceptions of using non-pharmacological interventions to manage their children's pain post-operatively and how it might be included in a qualitative SR or QES looking at parents' perceptions of managing their children's pain. Have a think what clinical guideline it might appear in, e.g. something like managing paediatric pain post-elective surgery that includes QES on children's and parent's preferences, perhaps?

Table 13.1 A summarisation of the EBP, SR, and clinical guideline development processes

Steps	EBP process	SR process	Clinical guideline process
PICOD PICO PEO	1. Pose a focused research question	1. Define an appropriate therapeutic question (PICOD/ PEO)	1. Define appropriate therapeutic **questions** (PICOD/ PEO) – up to 15
	2. Search for the evidence	2. Search the literature: Electronically and manually Published and unpublished English and non-English	2. Search the literature: Electronically and manually Published and unpublished English and non-English
	3. Critically appraise the evidence	3. Assess the **primary studies** for eligibility study quality: Reported findings	3. Assess the **systematic reviews** for eligibility study quality: Reported findings
✗ OR **✓**	4. Make a decision to implement the evidence (or not) alongside your clinical experience, patients' preferences, and resources	4. In an SR summarise the evidence in "evidence tables"; **compare the benefits and harms** Make a decision to implement the evidence (or not) alongside your clinical experience, patients' preferences (potentially informed by QES), and resources	4. In a clinical guideline summarise the evidence in "evidence tables"; **compare the benefits, harms, and costs** Make a decision to implement the evidence (or not) alongside your clinical experience, patients' preferences (potentially informed by QES), and resources
	5. Evaluate this	5. Evaluate this	5. Evaluate this

Critical appraisal of guidelines

Just as we have seen with primary research and SRs, critical appraisal of clinical guidelines is still necessary. The Appraisal of Guidelines for Research and Evaluation (AGREE) II Instrument (Brouwers et al, 2010) is a tool that assesses the methodological rigour and transparency in which a clinical guideline is developed. It includes 23 items which target various aspects of practice guideline quality.

Summary

- Remember in Chapter 1 we discussed that as well as clinical experience, research evidence must be incorporated into health care decision making. It is also important that patient preferences and resources be taken into account.
- We have seen that primary research feeds into systematic reviews, which feed into clinical guidelines.
- Clinical guidelines are crucial to inform appropriate cost-effective and efficient health care.
- Clinical guidelines are produced in a systematic and rigorous way.
- Quantitative SRs of RCTs are the main sources of evidence used to inform clinical guidelines regarding **"what works best"**.
- Recently Cochrane and NICE have joined forces to speed up this process.
- There have also been suggestions to use QES to answer a different sort of question related to **"how it makes people feel"** in order to inform patient preferences.
- This signals a move to in addition to wanting to know **"what works best"** when making clinical decisions, it also important to know **"how it makes people feel"**, although the methods are still evolving and the debates are still continuing.
- AGREE is an appraisal tool for clinical guidelines

References

Balshem H, Helfand M, Schunemann HJ, Oxman AD, Kunz R, Brozek J. et al. (2011) GRADE guidelines: 3. Rating the quality of evidence. *Journal of Clinical Epidemiology*; 64: 401–406.

Booth A. (2017) Qualitative evidence synthesis. In Facey K, Ploug Hansen H, Single A (Eds) *Patient Involvement in Health Technology Assessment* (pp. 187–199). Singapore: Adis. ISBN 9789811040689 QES and patient preferences

Brouwers MC, Kho ME, Browman GP, Burgers JS, Cluzeau F, Feder G, Fervers B, Graham ID, Grimshaw J, Hanna SE, Littlejohns P, Makarski J, Zitzelsberger L. (2010) AGREE II: Advancing guideline development, reporting, and evaluation in health care. *Preventive Medicine*; *51*(5): 421–424. ISSN 0091-7435. doi: 10.1016/j.ypmed.2010.08.005.

Carroll C. (2017) Qualitative evidence synthesis to improve implementation of clinical guidelines. *BMJ*; 356: j80. doi: 10.1136/bmj.j80

Glenton C, Lewin S, Norris SL. (2016) Chapter 15: Using evidence from qualitative research to develop WHO guidelines. In *Handbook for Guideline Development*. 2nd edn. Geneva: WHO.

Graham R, Mancher M, Wolman D. et al. (2011) *Clinical Practice Guidelines We Can Trust*. 1st edn. Washington, DC: The National Academics Press.

Hill J, Bullock I, Alderson P. (2011) A Summary of the methods that the National Clinical Guideline Centre uses to produce Clinical Guidelines for the National Institute for Health and Clinical Excellence. *Annals of Internal Medicine*; *154*: 752–757.

Howick J, Chalmers I, Glasziou P, Greenhalgh T, Heneghan C, Liberati A, Moschetti I, Phillips B, Thornton H. (2011) *Explanation of the 2011 Oxford Centre for Evidence-Based Medicine (OCEBM) Levels of Evidence (Background Document)*. Oxford Centre for Evidence-Based Medicine. www.cebm.net/index.aspx-?o=5653

Lewin S, Glenton C. (2018) Are we entering a new era for qualitative research? Using qualitative evidence to support guidance and guideline development by the World Health Organization. *International Journal for Equity in Health*; *17*(1): 126. doi: 10.1186/s12939-018-0841-x. PMID: 30244675

National Guideline Centre. (2021) www.rcplondon.ac.uk/about-us/what-we-do/national-guideline-centre-ngc. Accessed on 04/11/2021.

National Institute for Health and Care Excellence. (2018) *Developing NICE Guidelines: The Manual*. National Institute for Health and Care Excellence. www.nice.org.uk/guidelinesmanual. Accessed on 04/11/2021.

Polit DF, Beck CT. (2018) *Essentials of Nursing Research: Appraising Evidence for Nursing Practice*. 9th edn. Philadelphia: Wolters Kluwer.

Royal College of Paediatrics and Child Health. (2020) *Setting Standards for the Development of Clinical Guidelines in Paediatrics and Child Health*. 5th edn. April. https://www.rcpch.ac.uk/resources/clinical-guidelines-process-manual-setting-standards-development-clinical-guidelines?msclkid=87a899b5cf8c11ecbff7d0bdb5d7448f. Accessed on 12/10/2021.

Scottish Intercollegiate Guideline Network. (2011) *A Guideline Developers' Handbook*. Edinburgh: Scottish Intercollegiate Guideline Network.

Smith R. (1992) Audit & research. *BMJ*; *305*: 905–906.

14 Your role in all of this?

We started off this EBP journey highlighting the fact that high-quality evidence and research needs to be incorporated into clinical decision making to ensure we give (or get) the best care.

I hope by taking you through the steps from the production of primary research to its incorporation into systematic reviews, which then inform clinical guidelines to guide practice, you now have a much clearer understanding of going from evidence to practice. My experience of teaching it this way rather than as the "end user" of a clinical guideline is that it gives you a much greater critical awareness of how the guidance came about.

In the first chapter I said there are some big questions to ask yourselves regarding health care interventions:

HOW DO YOU KNOW IF THEY WORK?
IS ONE BETTER THAN ANOTHER?
HOW DOES THAT MAKE SOMEONE FEEL?
CAN YOU TRUST THE CLAIMS?
WHO ARE THE STAKEHOLDERS?
ARE THERE ANY ETHICAL IMPLICATIONS?
"RESEARCH SAYS . . ." DOES IT?
"THE EVIDENCE SUGGESTS . . ." DOES IT?

You are hopefully now in a better position, having appreciated the processes involved in EBP: constructing focused clinical research questions; developing your search skills to find evidence; identifying and interpreting different types of evidence relevant to what you need

DOI: 10.4324/9781003156017-18

to know; demonstrating competent skills in the appraisal of evidence, particularly the quantitative; describing, interpreting, and evaluating findings, again particularly the quantitative; and considering issues related to using this evidence to bring about practice change to know how to go about answering such questions.

Look at the steps I suggest you take in Table 14.1 as a good starting point to try to be an EB practitioner. I hope you find it helpful and that it is now more meaningful to you, having engaged with the material in the preceding chapters.

You may find that you can follow a "top-down" approach because there are lots of good-quality primary studies that have been systematically reviewed and fed into a clinical guideline already, which is great. You may find within the guideline that some practices have SRs of RCTs to underpin them, or a primary study, or expert consensus. There may be a QES to inform patient preferences. It will vary from topic to topic, guideline to guideline. Remember also to check how up-to-date it is.

Alternatively you may find you need to take a "bottom-up" approach, where you have scratched the surface and found there is no clinical guideline, or there are primary studies but they have not been systematically reviewed, or there are no primary studies at all. This is where you might find yourself signing up for a master's or a PhD course to carry out such SRs or primary research yourself! If that's not your thing, of course, there is great value in knowing how to try to be an evidence-based practitioner by following the EBP steps to develop yourself professionally.

Table 14.1 Steps you could take to be an evidence-based practitioner

Steps	*EBP process*
PICOD PICO PEO	1. Pose a focused research question If it is a "what works best", use PICOD If it is an "is there an association", use PICO If it is a "how does it feel", use PEO

(Continued)

Table 14.1 (Continued)

	2. Search for the evidence First look to see if there's a clinical guideline If no clinical guideline look to see if there's an SR For "what works best", look for a quantitative SR that has reviewed RCTs For an "is there an association", look for a quantitative SR that has reviewed cohort studies (or case-control studies) For a "how does it feel", look for a qualitative SR/QES that has reviewed qualitative studies If no systematic review look to see if there are pertinent primary studies For a "what works best", look for relevant RCTs For an "is there an association", look for cohort studies (or case-control studies) For a "how does it feel", look for primary qualitative studies
	3. Critically appraise the evidence To appraise a clinical guideline, use e.g. AGREE II To appraise an SR, use e.g. CASP tool for SR To appraise a quantitative RCT, use e.g. Cochrane ROB tool To appraise a quantitative NRS, use e.g. ROBiNRS tool To appraise a qualitative study, use e.g. CASP tool for qualitative study
✗ OR ✓	4. Make a decision to implement the evidence (or not) alongside your clinical experience, patients' preferences, and resources Consider the strength of the evidence: Clinical guideline SR: use e.g. GRADE or GRADE CERQual Primary study 5. Evaluate this using audit tool

Some other considerations:

- There are debates around what constitutes evidence.
- There are other types of quantitative research.
- There are other types of qualitative research.
- There are other types of systematic reviews.
- There are differences in views and tools for how best to appraise quantitative studies.
- There is empirical research looking into if there are worse sources of bias than others.
- In quantitative research, there is hypothesis testing and p values and estimation and confidence intervals and debates whether to report one or the other or both.
- There are differences in views and tools around how best to appraise qualitative studies.
- Primary and secondary research methods are still evolving.
- There are discussions around how quantitative data should be synthesised in quantitative systematic reviews.
- There are discussions around how qualitative data can be used in quantitative systematic reviews.
- There are discussions around how (and if) qualitative data should be synthesised in qualitative systematic reviews (QESs).
- There are discussions around how systematic reviews can be systematically reviewed!
- There are other guideline developers.
- There are other authors, initiatives, collaborations, and organisations instrumental in the EBP movement.

Evidence underpinning my practice

I feel with such a book I should mention what evidence underpins my practice as a teacher of EBP, since the EBP movement has also influenced the practice of educators.

As you saw in Chapter 1, in nursing and health care, professionals are encouraged to make decisions about practice based on their clinical experience, the research evidence, patients' preferences, and resources. As a teacher I have been influenced by my own education and experiences and the research evidence – especially SRs looking at the effectiveness of educational interventions, along with my students' preferences and resources.

In the 1990s when I began my teaching career, it was suggested that to produce EBP practitioners that would think critically and ask the pertinent health care questions and access, appraise, and analyse research, there needed to be a shift from "memorizing of facts to critical reasoning" (Glasziou et al, 2011, Greenhalgh, 1997, Rohwer et al, 2013). I was also influenced by Iain Chalmers, one of the cofounders of the Cochrane Collaboration, when I attended a clinical trials course in Edinburgh and had a brief chat after one of his presentations regarding the value and need to evaluate the effectiveness of nursing interventions. It inspired me to be involved in an RCT evaluating an alternating pressure mattress, then to be involved with Cochrane to undertake an SR evaluating topical negative pressure for chronic wounds. These experiences I hope helped underpin my teaching with content validity and credibility.

Some of the research was showing that interactive teaching was the most effective way of teaching EBP (Khan & Coomarasamy, 2006), but this just referred to lecture-based or face-to-face teaching. E-learning was just coming on board (Ruiz et al, 2006). E-learning was thought to have the advantage in that if adult learners were intrinsically motivated, it would shift the learning from "expert-led to user-led learning", as access to the educational materials could take place at "their own time, pace and place" (Clark, 2002, Ruggeri et al, 2013). However, a disadvantage potentially was thought to be social isolation and technical problems (Cook, 2007). This was probably still true for lecturers and students alike during the pandemic in 2021. An SR conducted by the World Health Organization (WHO) concluded that in terms of increasing EBP knowledge and skill acquisition, face-to-face and e-learning are as good as each other, but the primary studies included were judged to be at high risk of bias. A more recent SR (Rohwer et al, 2017) suggests that both used together to produce a blended approach are better at not only increasing EBP knowledge and skills but also attitudes and behaviour. Another recent overview of systematic reviews (Young et al, 2014) found that when comparing single interventions with multifaceted interventions, the latter were more likely to increase EBHC knowledge, skills, attitude, and behaviour. Feedback on specific goals in a timely manner also has a large impact on students' learning, which encouraged me to provide it formatively and summatively (Hattie & Timperley, 2007). These are the main reasons why I chose a blended approach (Liu et al, 2016) to teach research and EBP using both face-to-face and e-learning, lectures, tutorials, workshops, journal appraisal, and regular feedback. So far, that is how I have tried to use evidence to inform my teaching practice.

Of course, I have been heavily influenced by my students too – feedback is a two-way process. Entering a classroom and observing and listening to my students when trying to engage them with EBP and reading their module evaluations have been hugely informative. Going off their levels of engagement and suggestions, I have tried to appeal to different styles of learning by using text and pictures, explaining the "big" picture or the minutia, devising easy then more challenging activities, and taking feedback on what worked well and not so well – especially when delivering tricky topics. I have tried to capture some of that – and incorporate it into this book – but, of course, you will have to judge for yourselves if this book has helped you make sense of EBP. I hope it has.

Summary

- I have tried to tell you a "tidy story", as it is my experience when teaching this subject that students need a neat framework to hang their new knowledge on before appreciating the complexities.
- I have chosen to focus on the approaches, associated data collection and analysis methods, and tools my students have used or come across the most frequently to get you started on your EBP journey.
- My experience as a teacher has been that some students embrace qualitative research but shy away from the quantitative research, preferring the qualitative as it "feels closer to nursing". However, nurses administer lots of interventions and need to know **"what works best"**. Hence, the focus more heavily in this book on the value and place for RCTs and quantitative SRs in nursing.
- In addition, the learning outcomes of degree- and master's-level EBP and research modules often require nurses and health care students to not only demonstrate competence in developing

focused research questions and search skills to access relevant evidence but to also critically appraise both quantitative and qualitative primary and secondary research (SR) and to evaluate and interpret both quantitative and qualitative data in relation to decision making and practice change.

- Whilst I didn't go into great methodological and statistical detail, I hope I provided sufficient information for you to read and start to make sense of the quantitative primary and secondary approaches.

- Be pleased with yourself for coming this far and the understanding you have gained. But please don't stop there. There are many interesting developments and debates around these topics and much more to know.

- I hope you feel better placed now to handle the more in-depth comprehensive texts written about EBP by far greater academics than myself.

References

Clark D. (2002) Psychological myths in e-learning. *Medical Teacher*; 24(6): 589–604.

Cook D. (2007) Web-based learning: pros, cons and controversies. *Clinical Medicine*; 7(1): 37–42.

Glasziou PP, Sawicki PT, Prasad K, Montori VM. (2011) Not a medical course, but a life course. *Academic Medicine*, 86(11): e4. doi: 10.1097/ACM.0b013e3182320ec9

Greenhalgh TMF. (1997) Towards a competency grid for evidence-based practice. *Journal of Evaluation in Clinical Practice*; 3(2): 161–165.

Hattie J, Timperley H. (2007) The power of feedback. *Review of Educational Research*; 77(1): 81–112. doi: 10.3102/003465430298487

Khan KS, Coomarasamy A. (2006) A hierarchy of effective teaching and learning to acquire competence in evidenced-based medicine. *BMC Medical Education*; 6: 59. doi: 10.1186/1472-6920-6-5

Liu Q, Peng W, Zhang F, Hu R, Li Y, Yan W. (2016) The effectiveness of blended learning in health professions: Systematic review and meta-analysis. *Journal of Medical Internet Research*; 18(1). doi: 10.2196/jmir.4807

Rohwer A, Motaze NV, Rehfuess E, Young T. (2017) E-learning of evidence-based health care (EBHC) in healthcare professionals: A systematic review. *Campbell Systematic Reviews*; 4. doi: 10.4073/csr.2017.4

Rohwer A, Young T, van Schalkwyk S. (2013) Effective or just practical? An evaluation of an online postgraduate module on evidence-based medicine (EBM). *BMC Medical Education*; *13*: 77. doi: 10.1186/1472-6920-13-77

Ruggeri K, Farrington C, Brayne C. (2013) A global model for effective use and evaluation of e-learning in health. *Telemedicine Journal and e-Health*; *19*(4): 312–321. doi: 10.1089/tmj.2012.0175

Ruiz JM, Mintzer MJ, Leipzig RM. (2006) The impact on e-learning in medical education. *Academic Medicine*; *81*(3): 207–212.

Young T, Rohwer A, Volmink J, Clarke M. (2014) *What Are the Effects of Teaching Evidence-based Health Care (EBHC)?* https://pubmed.ncbi.nlm.nih.gov/24489771. Accessed on 20/10/2021.

Index

2 x 2 table ("honey") 89
2 x 2 table ("rapid heal") **84, 86, 89**
95% confidence interval: calculation 108, 113; interpretation **88, 90, 99, 101–102**

acronyms, usage 27
adult field example **15**
advanced clinical practitioner (ACP) question: answer, quantitative approach **44–45**; example **43–44**; "what works best" question **57**
advanced clinical practitioner (ACP) research interests, philosophies (application) 43
advanced nurse practitioner (ANP): PICO/PEO examples 30; research questions 43
advanced nurse practitioner (ANP) questions 19, **20–21**; search strategy, example **32**
alternative therapies (health care intervention) 1
analytic phase 39, **78**
AND (Boolean operator) 28
Applied Social Sciences Index and Abstracts (ASSIA) 26

Appraisal of Guidelines for Research and Evaluation (AGREE) II Instrument tool, usage 171
association 6, 17, 31, 66–70, 72–74, 105
asterisk symbol, usage 27
attrition bias 111; reduction **56, 62, 108**; risk 114

bias: appearance 55, **61**; appearance, consideration 60–61; approach 53–55; assessment, risk 108; attrition bias, reduction **56, 62, 108**; "bubbles" 54, 61; Cochrane Risk of Bias (ROB) tool 110–111; detection bias, reduction **56, 62, 108**; data analyst blindness 79; performance bias, risk **56, 61, 108**, 110–111; risk 111; selection bias, reduction **56, 61, 108**; sources 57, 65; sources, minimisation 65
bias minimisation 55, 77; RCT features, usage 55; steps **56, 61–62**
binary outcome 84
BIOSIS database **26**
blinding, impact **109**
Boolean operators, usage 28–32
bottom-up approach 174

Campbell Collaboration **149**
case-control approach **70**, **73**
case-control design **17**
case-control studies (quantitative)
   5, 8, 64; description **70–71**;
   example **72**; hypothetical **73–74**
cases: outcome, inclusion/exclusion
   71; researcher identification **70**
causation 6
cause and effect relationship,
   evidence **7**
CENTRAL **26**
child field example **16**
children's nurse question: answer,
   qualitative approach **46–47**;
   children's nurse "how does it feel"
   question **127**
children's nurse question/search
   strategy **46**
chronic wounds summary, "rapid
   heal" (hypothetical trial) **77–78**
citation indexes, evidence **26**
clinical audit 168
clinical decision making 4
clinical decisions,
   recommendations 164
clinical guidelines: critical
   appraisal 171; defining 164–165;
   draft guideline, production
   167; EBP clinical guidelines/
   implementation 164; final
   guideline, production 167–168;
   implementation 168; qualitative
   research, usage 168–169;
   quantitative research, usage 168;
   scope, preparation 166; steps 165;
   topic, referral 165
clinical guidelines development
   165–168; group, establishment
   166–167; processes,
   summarisation **170**
Cochrane, Archie **149**
Cochrane Collaboration 148, **149**,
   154–155, **156**
Cochrane Handbook 25

Cochrane Library: evidence **26**;
   need, reason 147
Cochrane Qualitative and
   Implementation Methods Group
   (CQRMG) 156, 158
Cochrane Risk of Bias (ROB)
   tool 110–111, 151; usage 111,
   113–115, 138
cohort approach, usage **68**
cohort studies 5, 64; description
   68–69; quantitative cohort
   studies 8
community health nurses:
   philosophies, application
   43; PICO/PEO examples
   30; questions 19; research
   questions 43
conceptual phase 39, **77**
constancy of conditions **52**,
   107
conference abstracts/proceedings,
   evidence **26**
confidence interval (CI) 87–90,
   105, 153, 154; 95% confidence
   interval, interpretation **88**, **90**,
   99, **101–102**; accounting 88, 99;
   calculation 98–99; examination
   98–100; formula 82; narrowing
   153; "no difference" interval,
   presence 82–83; usage 80–83
Confidence in the Evidence
   from Reviews of Qualitative
   Research (GRADE-CERQual)
   approach 160
consolidated criteria for reporting
   qualitative research (COREQ)
   document, features **139**
CONSORT 114; statement
   107–109
Consort document, features
   109–110
content analysis **121**
continuous data **97**
continuous measures, interpretation
   102

continuous outcomes **97**; effect measures 95
continuous quantitative data 105
control: need 65; reduction **74**; risk 84
control-gathering information, opportunity (reduction) **71**
counter-interventions **109**
critical appraisal process 37, 55, 76, 113, 141
Critical Appraisal Skills Programme (CASP) tool 112; application 112–113, 140–141; usage 113–115, 140; usage, process 141–142
critical theorists, thinking **42**
critical thinking, demonstration 142
Cumulative Index for Nursing and Allied Health (CINAHL) **26**

data: analysis 113, 141; credibility/ transferability/dependability/ confirmability **41**, **47**; existing data (qualitative data collection method) **120**; valid and reliable (quantitative data collection method) **40**, **45**, **67**
databases, search **26–27**, 29
data collection 45, 113, **123**; methods 120; phase 39, **78**; questions/prompts, usage **139**; semi-structured/unstructured in-depth interviews, usage 128, **136**
descriptive phenomenology, development **119**
descriptive phenomenology, steps **122–124**; application **127–129**, **136–137**
descriptive qualitative studies 120
design: hierarchy **5**; improvement, RCT features (usage) 55; non-randomised quantitative designs 64; phase **78**
"Design" logo 50, *118*

detection bias 111; risk 114
detection bias, reduction **56**, **62**, **108**; data analyst blindness 79, 96
dichotomous measures, interpretation **91**
dichotomous outcomes **83**, **84**; effect measures, defining 77
dichotomous quantitative data 105
difference measures 83, 95
discourse analysis **121**
dissemination phase 39, **78**
dissertations/theses, evidence **26**
district nurse (DN) questions 19, **30–31**; search strategy, example **30–31**
dressings (health care intervention) 1

educational interventions (health care intervention) 1
effect in time, effect (precession) 64
effectiveness: continuous measures, interpretation **102**; dichotomous measures, interpretation **91**; quantitative SRs 155
effect measures 79, 83–84, 95, 153; defining 77
e-learning 177, 178
Embase **26**
empirical phase **78**
estimation, confidence intervals (usage) 81–83
ethical approval **52**
ethnography 118, **139**; meta-ethnography **156**; similarities 119
EThOS **26**
evidence: appearance 5–8; hierarchy 5, 7, 148; inclusion, need **4**; need 7–8; quality, determination 37; search, location 25; search, places (list) **26–27**; search, process 25; understanding 2

evidence-based health care (EBHP) knowledge 177
evidence-based interventions 155
evidence-based medicine 3
evidence-based practice (EBP) 1, **149**; bottom-up approach 174; clinical guidelines/ implementation 164; defining 3; evidence 176–178; requirement 3; steps **8**, **13**; summarisation **170**
evidence-based practice (EBP) process 19; education 13; SR processes, similarities **159**
evidence-based practitioner: becoming, steps **174–175**; considerations 176; role 173
evidence-based public health 3
Evidence for Policy and Practice Information and coordination centre (EPPI-centre) 148, **149**
existing data (qualitative data collection method) **120**
experimental approach, usage **40, 44**
experiment, execution 82
exposed *71*
exposed cohort 69
extraneous variables, influence 64
extrinsic variables **52**

face-to-face learning 178
face-to-face teaching 177
findings, dissemination **40, 45, 47, 67, 68, 70, 73**
focused research question: assembly process 13; assembly process, framework (usage) 14; examples 14–19; Population, Exposure to, Outcome (PEO) structure, usage **18**; Population, Intervention, Counter-intervention, Outcome (PICO) structure, usage **15–17**; Population, Interest in, Outcome (PIO) structure, usage **18**; posing, steps 11

focus groups (qualitative data collection method) **120**
forest plot *153*; hypothetical forest plot **153**

general health care databases, evidence **26**
Goldacre, Ben **4**, **27**
Grading of Recommendations, Assessment, Development and Evaluations (GRADE) approach 160, 167
grey literature databases, evidence **26**
grounded theory 118, **120**, 139, 157; similarities 119
groups/interventions, difference (absence) 85, 98
guideline development groups (GDGs) 167
guidelines: critical appraisal 171; development group, establishment 166–167; draft guideline, production 167; final guideline, production 167–168; implementation 168; scope, preparation 166; topic, referral 165

healing, "rapid heal" effect (hypothetical trial) **84**
health care decision making 4
health care interventions 1, 149; questions 2
health care research, definition **37**
health visitor (HV) questions **20**; search strategy, example **31**
hermeneutics **119**
honey effectiveness, establishment (hypothetical trial) **44**
honey (effect), examination (hypothetical trial) **89, 100**
"Honey" RCT representation 60, *107*

"honey trial" hypothetical
106–107; Critical Appraisal
Skills Programme (CASP) tool,
application 112–113
"how does it feel": children's nurse
"how does it feel" question *127*;
consideration 29, **32**, **43**, **46**,
121; illumination **7**; question
12, **14**, **18–21**, **38**, 43, 126,
157; relationship **6**; researchers,
qualitative approach (usage) 118;
research question **41**, **47**
"how does that make someone feel"
question 1
"how someone feels": knowledge 5,
42; nursing questions **8**, **29**, **127**,
158; relationship 169
hypothesis testing, p values (usage)
80–81
hypothesis test, usage 83
hypothetical forest plot **153**, 154
hypothetical honey trial: inclusion,
consideration 169; results 151–152
hypothetical "parents' perceptions"
phenomenological study,
inclusion (consideration) 169
hypothetical "parents' perceptions"
study **46**, **127**, **135**
hypothetical qualitative systematic
review, consideration 157–158
hypothetical quantitative SR,
consideration 150–154
hypothetical RCT: features,
understanding 106; impact 100
hypothetical scenario, descriptive
phenomenology (application)
122–124, **136–137**
hypothetical systematic review
(hypothetical SR): hypothetical
honey trial, inclusion
(consideration) 169; hypothetical
"parents' perceptions"
phenomenological study,
inclusion (consideration) 169;
studies, results **152**

independent variable/intervention,
manipulation **67**
in-depth interviews (qualitative
data collection method) **120**;
usage **128**
inferential methods 80–83
interest, factor (measurement) **70**
interim analysis **109**
internal validity 5, 108
interpretive phenomenology
119, 157
interpretivists, thinking 41
interval estimate 99; calculation,
involvement 82
intervention/exposure, manipulation
(absence) **71**
interventions **109**; effectiveness,
establishment 64
intrinsic variables **52**
"is there a cause and effect":
question **15–16**; relationship,
nursing questions **7**, **28**, **88**
"is there an association": question 7,
17, **69–71**, 72, **73**; relationship,
nursing questions **7**, **72**

Joanna Briggs Institute 148, **156**
journals, evidence **26**

known variables, unknown variables
(balance) 65

learning disabilities field example **18**
lecture-based teaching 177
Lind, James **149**
low-level interpretation 121

mean difference (MD) 95–98,
100–101, 154; calculation 108,
113; interpretation **98**, **101**;
number line *100*, 102
measure (quantitative data
collection method) 52, 59, 78;
measuring instrument **40**; valid
and reliable **40**, **45**, **67**

medical devices (health care intervention) 1

medication (health care intervention) 1

Medline **26**

mental health field example **17**

meta-analysis 148

meta-ethnography **156**

methodological coherence **122**

Mills, John Stuart 64

narrative (analysis), qualitative framework (usage) **124, 128, 136**

National Guideline Centre, guidelines 165

National Health Service (NHS) guidelines, development 165

National Institute for Clinical Excellence (NICE) guidelines 164–165, 168

National Institute for Health and Care Excellence 165

National Institute for Health Research (NIHR) 168

national/international trial registers, evidence **27**

"no difference" value, presence 82–83

non-interrupted time series design **67**

non-pharmacological interventions 140, 142

non-randomised quantitative designs 64; existence 66

non-randomised studies (NRSs) 66, 74; critical appraisal 114–115; quantitative non-randomised studies (quantitative NRSs) 105

non-verbal communication 127

not exposed *71*

not exposed cohort 69

null hypothesis (NH) **51–53**; initiation 80; rejection 60, 80; result/difference, relationship 81; testing 80

number line, representation 88, *91*, *100*, 102

nurses: children's nurse question, answer (qualitative approach) **46–47**; children's nurse question/ search strategy **46**; district nurse (DN) questions **18**; health care intervention questions 2; thinking, shift 2; topics of interest, examples **38**

Nursing and Midwifery Council (NMC), nurse practise perspective **4**

nursing questions **7, 8**; "is there a cause and effect" relationship, nursing questions **7, 28, 88**; "is there an association" relationship, nursing questions **7, 72**

observation (qualitative data collection method) **120**; structured 40, 45

odds 86–87

odds of the event in the control group (O_C) 86

odds of the event in the experimental group (O_E) 86

odds ratio (OR) 86–87, 105; 2 x 2 table **86**

open-ended questionnaires (qualitative data collection method) **120**

OR (Boolean operator) 28

oral mucositis **45**, 61; 2 x 2 table **89**; hypothetical honey trial (bias risk), Cochrane ROB tool (usage) 114; presence 90; presence/absence, honey (effect) **89**

"other/extraneous variables," ruling out 64–65

outcome (O) **52**; binary outcome 84; dichotomous outcomes 84; dichotomous outcomes, effect measures (defining) 77; inclusion/ exclusion 69, *71*; pre-specified outcomes **109**; review outcome 160

parents' perception study (qualitative studies), CASP tool (application) 140–141
participants of interest, identification **123**, **128**, **136**
participants, random assignment **44–45**
performance bias: reduction **108**; risk **56**, 61, 110–111, 114
phenomenology 5, 118, **139**; definition 121; descriptive phenomenology, steps **122–124**; descriptive phenomenology, steps (application) **127–129**; similarities 119
philosophical underpinnings **44–45**
philosophical viewpoints **41–42**
planning phase **78**
plural/singular forms, usage 27
Point estimate 81–82
Population, Exposure to, Outcome (PEO) 14, 140, 157; framework, usage (demonstration) **29**; structure, usage **18**; table **18**
Population, Intervention, Counter-intervention, Outcome (PICO) 14, 53, 112; construction 89; structure, usage **15–17**
Population, Intervention, Counter-intervention, Outcome, Design (PICOD) **15**; framework, usage (demonstration) **28**; table **15–17**, **27**
Population, Interest in, Outcome (PIO) 14; structure, usage **18**
positivists, thinking **41**
post-positivists: perspective 125; thinking **42**
Preferred Reporting Items for SRs and Meta-analyses (PRISMA) statement 160
pre-specified outcomes **109**
presumed cause, presumed effect (empirical relationship) 64
psycho-social interventions (health care intervention) 1

psycINFO **26**
PubMed Central **26**
p values, usage 80–81

qualitative approach, usage **40**, **47**
qualitative data, analysis 41; approaches 120–121; methods **121**
qualitative data, collection methods **120**
qualitative designs 5; characteristics 118
qualitative evidence, critical appraisal 132
qualitative evidence synthesis (QES) 157–158, 168–169, 174
qualitative framework, usage **124**
qualitative quality criteria **125–126**, **129**; application **137–138**; steps **133–134**
qualitative research: description 118–119; questions, examples **14**; requirement 19; studies, appraisal 118; usage 168–169
qualitative research approach **119–120**; quantitative research approach, differences **6–7**; requirements **47**
qualitative scenario **40–41**, **46–47**
qualitative skills, Critical Appraisal Skills Programme (CASP) tool (usage) 140–141
qualitative studies **46**; CASP tool, application 138, 140; design **18**; reporting, improvement 138; systematic reviews 8
qualitative systematic reviews 156; hypothetical qualitative systematic review, consideration 157–158; milestones **156–157**
quantitative cohort studies 8; design **17**
quantitative data: analysis **40**, **45**, **67**; collection **40**, **45**, **67**; continuous quantitative data

105; dichotomous quantitative data 105

quantitative design 5; characteristics 50; consideration 64; non-randomised quantitative designs 64; randomised controlled trial 50; RCT quantitative design 64

quantitative evidence, critical appraisal process 105, 114–115

quantitative non-randomised studies (quantitative NRSs) 105

quantitative quality criteria **125–126**

quantitative randomised controlled trials (quantitative RCTs), characteristics 105

quantitative research: approaches, qualitative research approaches (differences) **6–7**; evidence 148; questions, examples **14**; usage 168

quantitative skills, Critical Appraisal Skills Programme (CASP) tool (usage) 112–113

quantitative scenario **39–40, 44–45**

quantitative systematic reviews 148; abstract, examination 154; hypothetical quantitative systematic review, consideration 150–154; milestones **149**; purposes, service 150150154

quasi-experiments (quantitative) 5, 64; description **67–68**

questions: advanced nurse practitioner (ANP) questions **20–21**; answering, evidence (search process) 25; district nurse (DN) questions **19**; focusing **15**; generation 13–19; health visitor (HV) questions **20**

questions (answering), evidence/ research (impact) 7–8

random allocation, absence 69, **71, 74**

randomisation, need 65

randomised controlled trial (RCT) 5, 16, 50; approach, usage **40, 44**; bias, appearance 55; bias "bubbles" 54, *61*; critical appraisal process 105; Critical Appraisal Skills Programme (CASP) tool 112; definition **51**; design **4**; execution 82; features, usage 55; "Honey" RCT representation 60; outcome 54, 60; quantitative design 64; quantitative randomised controlled trials (quantitative RCTs), characteristics 105; "rapid heal" RCT representation 53; steps **58–59**; steps, application **51–53**; strength 65; trial 51

"rapid heal" (RH): 2 x 2 table **84**; dressing 53, **56**, 83; effect, hypothetical trial **84**; example 81; experimental group 85–87; hypothetical trial **77–78**; RCT representation 53, 79, 96

ratio measures 83, 95

relative risk 84

research: agenda **150**; need 7–8; practice 1; purpose, statement **122, 127, 136**; quantitative/ qualitative research questions, examples **14**; trustworthiness 37; understanding 2

research hypothesis (RH): design **51**; formulation 80

research process: case-control study 70, 73; cohort study 68; 67qualitative 40, 46; quasi experiment 67; RCT, relationship 39, **44**; researcher guidance 39

research question: assembly process 13; example **40–41**

results, selective reporting 56–57

review outcome 160

risk/likelihood **85, 90**
Risk of Bias in NRS (ROBiNRS) tool 114
risk of the event in the control group (R_C) 84–85, 89
risk of the event in the experimental group (R_E) 84, 89
risk ratio (RR) 84–85, 87–89, 105, 153; 95% confidence interval 113; calculation 108, 150; interpretation **85, 90**; number line, representation 91; study **151–152**; value 87
risks 84–85
root words, variations 27

sample, selection **123, 128, 136**
sample size, confidence 65
scientific medicine **149**
scores, collation/analysis **52**
Scottish Intercollegiate Guideline Network (SIGN) 165
search 25; places, list **26–27**
search strategy: children's nurse question, answer (qualitative approach) **46–47**; children's nurse question/search strategy **46**; example **30–32, 43–44**; usage 30
search strategy, construction 30, 148; PICOD framework, usage (demonstration) **28**; Population, Exposure to, Outcome (PEO) framework, usage (demonstration) **29**; process 27–28
selection bias 111; reduction **56, 61, 108**; risk 114
semi-structured in-depth interviews, usage 128, **136**
"setting the scene" 42
source articles 26
specialist community public health nurses: philosophies, application 43; PICO/PEO examples

30; questions 19; research questions 43
spelling variations 27
stakeholders, interest 166
Standards for Reporting Qualitative Research (SRQR), development 138
statistical analysis **110**
statistical constructs, defining 95
statistical evaluation, interval estimate calculation (involvement) 82
stopping guidance **109**
STROBE statement 114
structured observation and measurement (quantitative data collection method) **40, 45**
study design, decision 51, 58, **122, 127**
subject-specific databases, evidence **26**
sudden infant death syndrome (SIDS): case-control study example **72**; hypothetical case-control study **73–74**
supporting quotations, providing **139**
synonyms, usage 27
systematic error 114
systematic reviewers: interest 157; studies, usage **151**
systematic reviews (SRs) 5; hypothetical quantitative SR, consideration 150–154; initiatives, need (reason) 147; process, EBP processes (similarities) **159**; process, steps 158–160; qualitative studies, SRs 8; quantitative systematic reviews 148; quantitative systematic reviews, milestones **149**; quantitative systematic reviews, purposes (service) **150**; summarisation **170**; systematic approach, usage 148

talking therapies (health care intervention) 1
textual analysis **121**
thematic analysis **121**
theoretical framework, decision **122**, **127**, **136**
theory triangulation 142
thick descriptions, absence 142
thinking, shift **2**
topical agents (health care intervention) 1
topical negative pressure (TNP) 14, 27, **38**; effect **39**
topics of interest, examples **38**
trial results registers, evidence **27**

unpublished/ongoing studies, evidence **27**

unstructured in-depth interviews, usage 128, **136**

values, range 82
variables: control 77; exposure **71**
visual analogue (VA) scale 100

Web of Science **26**
"what works best" 15–16; consideration 28; decision making 155; knowledge 5, 148; relationship **6**
"what works best" questions 7, 19, 43, 57, **57**, 77, **156**; commonness **1**
wild cards 27
World Health Organization (WHO): evidence 168; SR, conducting 177